CARDIOLOGY

#1

Inappropriate shocks occur in 20 to 25% of those with an AICD in place. The most common cause of an inappropriate shock is:

A. Lead fracture

B. Loud electrical noise

C. Atrial Fibrillation

D. Inappropriate sensing

E. Sudden body movements

The Kaji Review

Emergency Medicine Clinical Review Book

Vol 1 Part 1

Amy H. Kaji, MD, PhD
Associate Professor of Clinical Medicine
Harbor-UCLA Medical Center
Department of Emergency Medicine

Daniel G. Ostermayer, MD
Assistant Professor of Emergency Medicine
University of Texas Health Science Center at Houston
Department of Emergency Medicine

ASSOCIATE EDITORS

Ami Yamamoto, MD
Harbor-UCLA Medical Center
Department of Emergency Medicine

Kevin P. Beres, DO
University of Texas Health Science Center at Houston
Department of Emergency Medicine

Silas Chiu MD, MS
Harbor-UCLA Medical Center
Department of Emergency Medicine

ASSISTANT EDITOR

Manpreet Singh, MD
Harbor-UCLA Medical Center
Department of Emergency Medicine

The Kaji Review

Welcome to the Kaji Review. This book is intended for students, residents, advanced practitioners, and senior physicians alike. Although formatted as a question book, the Kaji Review is really an evidence based clinical case book to advance your bedside knowledge with 774 questions.

We hope you will use this question book to improve clinical care and encourage lifelong learning. Content pulls heavily from textbooks and LLSA readings. Topics are focused on emergency care but also cover outpatient and inpatient medical and surgical topics. Sometimes questions will have more than one correct answer, just like our patients. Don't worry, we will give you a hint on those.

Often the explanations include textbook references, evidence based guidelines, online resources, and specific details of clinical research. If we could find a full text or appropriate video or illustration we included links. Questions are grouped by section so you can focus on specific topics and dive deeply into relevant clinical content.

#1

Answer: C

The incidence of inappropriate ICD firing is reported to occur in 20 - 25% of patients, with the main cause being atrial fibrillation. The reported percentages for inappropriate shocks are:

A. Atrial fibrillation (44%)
B. Supraventricular tachycardia (36%)
C. Abnormal sensing (20%).

Other less common causes include electrical noise, inappropriate sensing, and ICD malfunction, such as lead fracture. Patients with supraventricular tachycardias (SVT) often experience more than one discharge. Dual chamber devices can reduce the frequency of inappropriate shocks, in which an atrial sensing lead can differentiate atrial tachycardia vs atrial flutter or fibrillation. Other settings, such as antitachycardia pacing, help to further discriminate atrial from ventricular dysrhythmias. Alternative methods for decreasing inappropriate shocks and atrial dysrhythmias include antiarrhythmic drugs and catheter ablation.

- *Daubert, et al. Inappropriate Implantable Cardioverter Defibrillator Shocks in MADIT II. 2008; 1357–65. full text*

- *Mitchell AR. Effect of atrial antitachycardia pacing treatments in patients with an atrial defibrillator: randomised study comparing subthreshold and nominal pacing outputs. Heart. 2002 May;87(5):433-7. full text*

#2

Which of the following patients/conditions has the lowest risk of bacterial endocarditis?

A. Patient with a prosthetic heart valve

B. Patient with a complex cyanotic congenital heart defect

C. Patient who has had a systemic-to-pulmonary shunt

D. Patient with an isolated atrial septal defect

E. Patient with a previous episode of endocarditis

#2

Answer: D

Patients with cardiac lesions that produce turbulent blood flow are predisposed to bacterial endocarditis, since there is greater risk of endothelial damage and vegetation formation. Cardiac conditions carrying the greatest risk are:

1. Ventricular septal defects
2. Aortic valvular stenosis
3. Tetralogy of Fallot
4. Single ventricular states
5. Prosthetic valves
6. Cardiac shunting procedures.

Atrial septal defects carry a low risk for endocarditis since atrial flow is much lower than ventricular flow and valvular flow. This decreases the risk of endothelial and valvular damage.

. *Rosen's Emergency Medicine 8th edition. 2013. Chapter 83: Infective Endocarditis and Valvular Heart Disease. 1106 - 1112.*

#3

Which of the following strategies has NOT been associated with shorter door-to-balloon times?

A. Prehospital ECG and activation of catheterization laboratory en route

B. Emergency department activation of the catheterization laboratory without routine cardiology consultation

C. Prompt feedback from data monitoring

D. Establishing a single call system to activate the entire catheterization laboratory team

E. Establishing a requirement that the cardiac catheterization team arrives within 60 to 90 minutes after being paged

#3

Answer: E

Establishing an expectation that team members arrive within 20-30 minutes after being paged is one of the strategies that has been associated with shorter door-to-balloon times. Other strategies include the following:

1. Prehospital ECG and activation of the catheterization laboratory en route
2. Direct transfer to the catheterization laboratory by emergency medical services using prehospital ECGs
3. Establishing emergency department guidelines and protocols for rapidly obtaining ECGs in triage
4. ED activation of catheterization laboratory without cardiology consultation
5. Single call activation of the catheterization laboratory
6. Prompt data feedback
7. Commitment from senior management and administration.

. *LLSA 2009: Brahmajee K, et al. Time to treatment in primary percutaneous intervention. N Eng J Med. 2007; 357:1631-1638. full text*

#4

Regarding acute myocardial infarction, when patients with normal and non-diagnostic electrocardiograms were compared with patients who had diagnostic electrocardiograms, patients with normal and non-diagnostic electrocardiograms had an in-hospital mortality that was:

A. Lower

B. Higher

C. The same

#4

Answer: A

Welch, et al. compared the in-hospital mortality among patients with AMI who had normal or nonspecific initial ECGs to patients with diagnostic ECGs. The multicenter study involved 391,208 patients with acute myocardial infarction who had an ECG that was normal (n = 30,759), nonspecific (n = 137,574), or diagnostic (n = 222,875). Diagnostic ECGs were defined as ST-segment elevation or depression and/or left bundle-branch block. They demonstrated in-hospital mortality rates of 5.7% (normal ECG), 8.7% (nonspecific ECG), and 11.5% (diagnostic ECG). The composite rates of mortality and life-threatening adverse events were 19.2% (normal ECG), 27.5% (nonspecific ECG), and 34.9% (diagnostic ECG).

After adjusting for other predictor variables, the odds of mortality for the normal ECG group was 0.59 (95% confidence interval [CI], 0.56-0.63; P<.001) and for the nonspecific group was 0.70 (95% CI, 0.68-0.72; P<.001), compared with the diagnostic ECG group. In this cohort, patients with normal or nonspecific ECGs had a lower in-hospital mortality than those with diagnostic ECGs.

- *LLSA 2006: Welch RD, et al. Prognostic value of a normal or nonspecific initial ECG in acute myocardial infarction. JAMA. 2001; 286: 1977-1984. full text*

#5

Acute symptoms of myocardial infarction (AMI) or prodromal symptoms occurring 1 month prior to the MI in women include all EXCEPT:

A. Fatigue

B. Shortness of breath

C. Weakness

D. Loss of consciousness

E. Sleep disturbances

#5

Answer: D

The most frequent prodromal symptoms experienced by women more than 1 month before AMI were:

- Fatigue (70.7%)
- Sleep disturbance (47.8%)
- Shortness of breath (42.1%).

Only 29.7% reported chest discomfort, a classic symptom in men.

The most frequent acute symptoms in women were:

- Shortness of breath (57.9%)
- Weakness (54.8%)
- Fatigue (42.9%)

Acute chest pain was absent in 43%.

- *LLSA 2006: McSweeney JC, et al. Women's early warning symptoms of acute myocardial infarction. Circulation. 2003; 108: 2619 -2623. full text*

#6

Which of the following is the LEAST helpful feature for increasing the probability that heart failure is the etiology of dyspnea?

A. Past history of heart failure

B. Paroxysmal nocturnal dyspnea

C. The sign of a third heart sound

D. The sign of a fourth heart sound

E. Electrocardiogram demonstrating atrial fibrillation

#6

Answer: D

Wang, et al. evaluated the usefulness of history, physical exam, and diagnostic tests in diagnosing heart failure. Below are the likelihood ratios of the various diagnostic characteristics and tests.

<u>**Positive predictors:**</u>

Past history of heart failure:

- Positive LR = 5.8; 95% CI, 4.1-8.0

Symptom of paroxysmal nocturnal dyspnea

- Positive LR = 2.6; 95% CI, 1.5-4.5

Sign of the third heart sound (S3) gallop

- Positive LR = 11; 95% CI, 4.9-25.0

Pulmonary venous congestion on X-ray

- Positive LR = 12.0; 95% CI, 6.8-21.0

Electrocardiogram showing atrial fibrillation

- Positive LR = 3.8; 95% CI, 1.7-8.8

Negative predictors:

Absence of a past history of heart failure

- Negative LR = 0.45; 95% CI, 0.38-0.53

Absence of dyspnea on exertion

- Negative LR = 0.48; 95% CI, 0.35-0.67

Absence of rales

- Negative LR = 0.51; 95% CI, 0.37-0.70

Absence of a cardiomegaly on chest radiograph

- Negative LR = 0.33; 95% CI, 0.23-0.48

Absence of electrocardiogram abnormality

- Negative LR = 0.64; 95% CI, 0.47-0.88

Serum B-type natriuretic peptide <100 pg/mL

- Negative LR = 0.11; 95% CI, 0.07-0.16

The authors conclude that for dyspneic adult emergency department patients, a directed history, physical examination, chest radiography, and electrocardiography should be performed. If the diagnosis of heart failure is still uncertain, a serum BNP level may be helpful.

- *LLSA 2007: Wang CS, et al. Does this Dyspneic patient in the emergency department have congestive heart failure? JAMA. 2005; 294(15):1944-1956. full text*

#7

Studies have shown that nesiritide provides symptomatic relief in patients with acutely decompensated heart failure compared to placebo. When comparing nesiritide with standard diuretic and vasodilator therapies, nesiritide may:

A. Improve creatinine clearance

B. Be associated with an increased risk of 30-day death

C. Be associated with a decreased risk of 30-day death

D. None of the above

#7

Answer: B

Sackner-Bernstein et al. performed a meta-analysis of trials evaluating nesiritide for the treatment of decompensated heart failure. Death within 30 days tended to occur more often among patients randomized to nesiritide therapy (35 [7.2%] of 485 vs 15 [4.0%] of 377 patients; risk ratio, 1.74; 95% CI, 0.97-3.12).

Compared with diuretic and vasodilator therapy, nesiritide may be associated with increased risk of death in the treatment of acutely decompensated heart failure.

- *LLSA 2007: Sackner-Bernstein JD, et al. Short-term risk of death after treatment with Nesiritide for decompensated heart failure. JAMA. 2005; 293: 1900-1905. full text*

#8

A 60 year old male who has an ICD in place presents in cardiac arrest. All of the following are appropriate management steps, EXCEPT:

A. Focus on treating potentially reversible causes of electromechanical dissociation (EMD) and Ventricular Fibrillation (VF)/Ventricular Tachycardia (VT)

B. Generally follow ACLS protocols.

C. Place the defibrillator pads directly over the device

D. Perform chest compressions in the standard fashion

E. After successful resuscitation, you should focus on the causes of ICD failure (electrolyte imbalance, myocardial ischemia or infarction, drug effects) that may be treated without ICD reprogramming or surgery.

#8

Answer: C

The most common causes of sudden death in patients with ICDs are:

- Electromechanical dissociation (EMD) after ICD conversion of VF or VT (29%)
- Defibrillator failure (25%) -VT or VF that was not terminated by the ICD shocks
- EMD not involving VF or VT (16%)
- Recurrent VF after successfully defibrillation (13%).

When treating a patient with an ICD in cardiac arrest, emphasis should be placed on external counter shocks and correcting all potentially reversible causes. Resuscitation should follow ACLS protocols. Most ICDs analyze and shock VF or VT within 30 seconds, so it should be assumed that a patient who presents with VF or VT has ICD failure. The external defibrillator pads should not be placed directly over the device, but rather, positioned anteroposteriorly.

- *Mitchell LB, et al. Sudden death in patients with implantable cardioverter defibrillators: the importance of post-shock electromechanical dissociation. J Am Coll Cardiol. 2002; Apr 17;39(8):1323-8. full text*

#9

Which of the following statements about pacemakers is TRUE?

A. The absence of ST segment elevations and T wave changes in a patient with a pacemaker rules out ischemia and infarction.

B. Right ventricular pacemakers produce a right bundle branch block.

C. Using Sgarbossa's Criteria on a paced patient or patient with a LBBB has poor sensitivity but high specificity for the diagnosis of STEMI.

D. High voltage electrical machinery has no risk of altering pacemaker function.

E. The most common cause of failure to capture (the absence of ventricular or atrial depolarization after a pacemaker spike) is hyperkalemia.

#9

Answer: C

Right ventricular pacemakers produce a left bundle branch (LBBB) pattern of depolarization, and thus, the ECG diagnosis of myocardial ischemia and infarction may be difficult. The Sgarbossa Criteria_has a low sensitivity but high specificity in evaluating a patient with a LBBB. In general, everyday electrical utilities and computers will not interfere with a pacemaker, although high voltage industrial machinery may offer some interference risk. The most common cause of non-capture is pacemaker lead dislodgment, which typically occurs within a few weeks of implantation. Other mechanical causes include insulation breaks and lead fractures.

- *Klimczak A, et al. Electrocardiographic diagnosis of acute coronary syndromes in patients with left bundle branch block or paced rhythm. Cardiol J. 2007; 14(2) 207-13. full text*

- *Shlipak MG, et al. Should the electrocardiogram be used to guide therapy for patients with left bundle-branch block and suspected myocardial infarction? JAMA. 1999; 281(8):714. full text*

#10

In the patient with an acute myocardial infarction and cardiogenic shock, which of the following constitutes optimal therapy?

A. Ensure adequate ventilation and oxygenation

B. Treat emergent arrhythmias

C. Administer aspirin if not aspirin allergic

D. Arrange for emergent PCI

E. All of the above

#10

Answer: E

All of the above would be indicated, and consideration should be given for inotropic agents. Evidence from randomized trials suggests that emergent revascularization improves mortality rates at 6 months and at one year.

- *Rosen's Emergency Medicine - Concepts and Clinical Practice. 8th edition. 2013. Chapter 78: Acute Coronary Syndrome. 997-1033.*

#11

What is the only post-return of spontaneous circulation intervention that has been shown to improve survival and functional outcome of comatose cardiac arrest survivors?

A. Transvenous pacing

B. Transcutaneous pacing

C. Intra-aortic balloon counterpulsation

D. Induced hypothermia

E. Inotropic agents

#11

Answer: D

Therapeutic hypothermia has been shown to improve survival and functional outcome in prospective randomized controlled trials. Although there are no absolute contraindications to hypothermia, relative contraindications include

1. Persistent dysrhythmias
2. Uncontrolled hemorrhage
3. Preexisting coagulopathy
4. Pregnancy
5. Drug overdose or status epilepticus causing coma
6. Terminal illness and a do-not-resuscitate order.

Patients who have received thrombolytics can still undergo hypothermia protocol. Recent evidence also suggests that traditional (32-34°C) cooling may be no better than 36°C. The main benefit from cooling may be the result of preventing fever.

- *Rosen's Emergency Medicine - Concepts and Clinical Practice. 8th edition. 2013. Chapter 83: Brain Resuscitation. 84-86.*
- *Nielsen N, et al. Targeted Temperature Management at 33°C versus 36°C after Cardiac Arrest. The New England Journal of Medicine. 2013; 369(23):2197-2206. full text*

#12

Which of the following statements is FALSE regarding the combined administration of epinephrine and vasopressin in cardiac arrest?

A. Animal studies suggest a benefit of combining vasopressin and epinephrine in cardiac arrest.

B. Human studies demonstrate no significant difference in survival to hospital admission.

C. Human studies demonstrate a significant benefit in return of spontaneous circulation.

D. Human studies demonstrate no significant difference in survival to hospital discharge.

E. Human studies demonstrate no significant difference in good neurologic recovery at the time of hospital discharge.

#12
Answer: C

Despite animal studies suggesting a benefit of combining vasopressin and epinephrine in cardiac arrest, this has never been confirmed in human studies. In a multicenter double-blind placebo-controlled trial of 2,894 patients in France, there were no differences in any of the primary or secondary outcomes between epinephrine alone or combined with 40 IU of vasopressin. These included survival to hospital admission or discharge, return of spontaneous circulation, or neurologic recovery at the time of hospital discharge. That being said, epinephrine in cardiac arrest has not been shown to have any mortality benefit, although it increases the rate of return of spontaneous circulation.

- *Gueugniaud PY, et al. Vasopressin and epinephrine vs. epinephrine alone in cardiopulmonary resuscitation. N Engl J Med. 2008; 359: 21. full text*
- *Hagihara A, et al. Prehospital epinephrine use and survival among patients with out-of-hospital cardiac arrest. JAMA. 2012; 307(11):1161-8. full text*

#13

Regarding the San Francisco Syncope Rules (SFSR), which of the following is FALSE?

A. The rule is based on five predictor variables.

B. One predictor variable is a history of CHF.

C. One predictor variable is a hematocrit below 30%.

D. Other predictor variables include an abnormal ECG, SBP < 90 mm Hg and shortness of breath.

E. The SFSR has been validated in multiple settings and populations.

#13

Answer: E

Birnbaum, et al. performed a prospective validation trial of the San Francisco syncope rule with 713 patients. The SFSR predicted a "serious seven day outcome" in only 45 out of 61 patients, and was falsely positive in 278 patients who had no serious outcome. Overall sensitivity was 74% and specificity was 57%. The 16 serious outcomes not predicted by the rule included one death, 8 ventricular arrhythmias, three strokes, and one SAH. Needless to say, the rule was not validated.

San Francisco Syncope Rule Criteria:

1. Congestive Heart Failure
2. Hematocrit < 30%
3. ECG abnormality
4. Shortness of breath
5. Systolic BP < 90 mmHg at triage.

- *Birnbaum A, et al. Failure to validate the San Francisco syncope rule in an independent emergency department population. Ann Emerg Med. 2008; 52: 151.*

- *MD Calc http://www.mdcalc.com/san-francisco-syncope-rule-to-predict-serious-outcomes/*

#14

A 58 year old male with dilated ischemic cardiomyopathy presents with dyspnea at rest and on exertion, and orthopnea. The X-ray demonstrates pulmonary edema, the ECG is unchanged from a previous ECG, and the pulse oximetry is 92% on a non-rebreather mask. After administration of nitrates, what is the best next step in management?

A. Endotracheal intubation

B. Digoxin

C. Nesiritide

D. Noninvasive ventilation

E. Albuterol nebulizer treatments

#14

Answer: D

In a systematic review of fifteen trials, noninvasive ventilation significantly reduced the mortality rate by nearly 45% compared with conventional therapy (risk ratio [RR], 0.55; 95% CI, 0.40-0.78; P = 0.72 for heterogeneity). The results were significant for continuous positive airway pressure, CPAP, (RR, 0.53; 95% CI, 0.35-0.81) but not for bilevel noninvasive pressure support ventilation, NIPSV, (RR, 0.60; 95% CI, 0.34-1.05), although there were fewer studies in the NIPSV group.

Both modalities showed a significant decrease in the intubation rates compared with conventional therapy. Although the level of evidence is higher for CPAP, there are no significant differences in clinical outcomes when comparing CPAP vs NIPSV.

- *LLSA 2009: Masip J, et al. Noninvasive ventilation in acute cardiogenic pulmonary edema: systematic review and meta-analysis. JAMA. 2005 Dec 28; 294(24): 3124-30. full text*

#15

A 57 yo male patient is found to have a Type B aortic dissection by CT and is still complaining of severe chest pain. While awaiting evaluation by the vascular surgery service, which of the following would be the LEAST appropriate treatment you could provide this patient with a BP of 190/100 and a HR of 100 bpm:

A. Opioids

B. Esmolol alone

C. Nitroprusside alone

D. Esmolol and Nitroprusside

E. Labetalol

#15

Answer: C

Early therapy for aortic dissection is directed towards two goals:

1. Reduction of blood pressure
2. Decrease the rate of rise of the arterial pulse (dP/dt) to diminish shearing forces.

First line therapy is the use of beta-blockers. Esmolol or labetalol can be administered as boluses and then maintained as an infusion with a target heart rate of 60 bpm and SBP 100-120 mmHg. Opioids should be administered in adequate amounts for pain control and to decrease sympathetic tone. Nitroprusside is a potent preload and afterload reducing agent that causes vasodilatation and arteriolar dilatation. Because vasodilators like nitroprusside can increase the heart rate and therefore increase dP/dt (increasing shearing force), a beta blocker should be started before or in conjunction with nitroprusside.

- *Rosen's Emergency Medicine - Concepts and Clinical Practice. 8th edition. 2013. Chapter 85: Aortic Dissection. 1127-1128.*
- *EmCrit - Aortic Dissection http://emcrit.org/podcasts/aortic-dissection/*
- *Kodama K, et al. Tight heart rate control reduces secondary adverse events in patients with type B acute aortic dissection. Circulation. 2008 Sep 30; 118(14 Suppl):S167-70. full text*

#16

Which of the following is NOT consistent with Dressler's syndrome?

A. Fever

B. Pleuritis and pleural effusion

C. Leukocytosis

D. Friction rub

E. Mediastinitis

#16

Answer: E

Dressler's syndrome is characterized by chest pain, fever, and pleural effusions. It is thought to be an immunologic reaction that occurs 2 to 6 weeks post MI. Aspirin or indomethacin is the standard therapy. An acute pericarditis 2-7 days following transmural MIs can also occur. It is manifested by low grade fever and a transient friction rub that is generally short-lived and disappears within 1-3 days of initiating aspirin treatment.

- *Rosen's Emergency Medicine - Concepts and Clinical Practice. 8th edition. 2013. Chapter 82: Pericardial and Myocardial. 1093.*

#17

Regarding pericardial disease, which of the following statements is FALSE:

A. Most cases of pericarditis are idiopathic.

B. Classic symptoms of pericarditis include chest pain, pericardial friction rub and ECG abnormalities including electrical alternans.

C. Pericardial effusion of less than 200cc usually will not produce cardiomegaly on chest X-ray.

D. Cardiac tamponade is the result of compression of the myocardium and increased pericardial pressure leading to decreased cardiac output.

E. Ventricular dysrhythmias are common in pericardial disease.

#17

Answer: E

Pericarditis has multiple causes that include infectious, post procedural, metabolic, neoplastic, and systemic connective tissue disorders. Ventricular dysrhythmias should not be caused by pericarditis. If they do occur in a patient diagnosed with pericarditis, the patient either has a concomitant myocarditis or intrinsic cardiac disease.

Patients with pericarditis generally recover fully after 3 weeks. The ECG will evolve over that time. The ECG stages are:

1. Diffuse ST segment elevation with possibility for concurrent PR depression
2. ST and PR segments become isoelectric and T wave flattening occurs
3. Deep symmetric T wave inversions
4. Normalization of T waves.

- *Rosen's Emergency Medicine - Concepts and Clinical Practice. 8th edition. 2013. Chapter 82: Pericardial and Myocardial. 1091-1093.*

#18

Vasodilatory agents would be the LEAST appropriate initial therapy in which of the following patients with chronic valvular disease?

A. Patient with chronic mitral and aortic insufficiency with a BP of 150/87 and CHF

B. Patient with mitral stenosis, BP of 137/70 and pink sputum

C. Patient with critical aortic stenosis with a BP of 120/45 and chest pain

D. Patient with mitral insufficiency with a BP of 180/90 and CHF

#18

Answer: C

Chronic valvular disease is commonly associated with CHF (most commonly mitral insufficiency and aortic stenosis). Patients with decompensated aortic stenosis have a fixed lesion and without adequate preload, they will become hypotensive. Generally vasodilators such as nitroglycerine should be avoided.

- *Rosen's Emergency Medicine - Concepts and Clinical Practice. 8th edition. 2013. Chapter 82: Pericardial and Myocardial Disease. 1078-1079.*

#19

Regarding pericardial disease, which of the following is FALSE?

A. ECG changes associated with pericarditis include ST elevation in all leads, except avR and V1.

B. To help distinguish the ST elevation of pericarditis from repolarization abnormality, take the ST elevation/T wave amplitude ratio. If the ratio is < 0.25, then it is more likely to be pericarditis, rather than early repolarization.

C. Patients may complain of retrosternal pain radiating to the trapezius ridge with pericarditis, which is improved with sitting forward.

D. The American College of Cardiology (ACC) and AHA recommend echocardiogram to rule out associated pericardial effusion in patients suspected of having pericarditis.

E. Consider admission for patients with pericarditis, particularly if they are immunocompromised, on warfarin, have an associated effusion, or have had significant chest trauma.

#19

Answer: B

The major clinical manifestations of acute pericarditis include:

1. Chest pain,
2. Pericardial friction rub
3. ECG changes — new diffuse ST elevation or PR depression
4. Pericardial effusion.

Absence of pericardial effusion does not exclude pericarditis. The normal early repolarization variant is often confused with acute pericarditis. It is characterized by ST elevation of the J point, which represents the junction between the end of the QRS complex (termination of depolarization) and the beginning of the ST segment (onset of ventricular repolarization). As a result, there is elevation of the ST segment itself, which maintains its normal configuration. ST elevation is most often present in the mid to lateral chest leads (V3-V6), although many leads can be involved.

Two findings that strongly favor pericarditis are PR depression and evolution of the ST and T changes, neither of which is seen in early repolarization. There can also be ST depression and PR elevation in leads aVR and V1.

In a prospective study, the most reliable distinguishing feature was the ratio of ST elevation to T wave amplitude in lead V6. If the ratio exceeds 0.25, acute pericarditis was present (positive and negative predictive values were both 100%).

- *Ginzton LE, Laks MM. The differential diagnosis of acute pericarditis from the normal variant: new electrocardiographic criteria. Circulation. 1982. May; 65(5): 1004-1009. full text*

- *Spodick DH. Differential characteristics of the electrocardiogram in early repolarization and acute pericarditis. N Engl J Med. 1976. 295(10): 523-526.*

#20

Which of the following statements regarding B-type Natriuretic Peptide (BNP) is FALSE?

A. Normal BNP levels increase with age

B. Normal BNP levels are higher in women

C. BNP levels are more accurate in obese patients

D. BNP levels are elevated in renal failure

#20

Answer: C

Normal plasma BNP values increase with age and are higher in women than men. Obese patients tend to have lower plasma BNP while patients with renal failure have elevated BNP.

- *Mehra MR, et al. Obesity and suppressed B-type natriuretic peptide levels in heart failure. J Am Coll Cardiol. 2004; 43: 1590. full text*

- *Redfield MM, et al. Plasma brain natriuretic peptide concentration: impact of age and gender. J Am Coll Cardiol. 2002; 40: 976. full text*

#21

Regarding hypertension in the ED, which of the following statements are TRUE?

A. ED blood pressure readings are accurate and reliable for screening asymptomatic patients for hypertension, but it is recommended that 2 separate measurements are obtained.

B. In addition to history and physical examination, screening for target organ damage in an asymptomatic patient may include urinalysis, serum creatinine level, ECG, and chest radiography.

C. There is no published evidence demonstrating improved patient outcomes or decreased mortality or morbidity with acute management of asymptomatic elevated blood pressure in the ED.

D. When ED treatment for asymptomatic hypertension is initiated, blood pressure management should attempt to gradually lower blood pressure and should not be expected to be normalized during the initial ED visit.

E. All of the above

#21

Answer: E

Much practice variation exists regarding the appropriate treatment of patients found to have asymptomatic hypertension in the ED. The ACEP clinical policy provides guidance to the provider but ultimately suggests that workup and therapy should be individualized. If there is concern for end organ dysfunction, consider obtaining an ECG and measuring the creatine. The patient without symptoms can have gradual blood pressure lowering as an outpatient with decisions to start a new antihypertensive or adjustment of current medications individualized to the patient. There are no specific target blood pressures that need to be achieved prior to patient discharge.

- *Wolf SJ, et al. Clinical policy: critical issues in the evaluation and management of adult patients in the emergency department with asymptomatic elevated blood pressure. Ann Emerg Med. 2013 Jul; 62(1):59-68. full text*

- *Decker WW, et al. Clinical policy: critical issues in the evaluation and management of adult patients with asymptomatic hypertension in the emergency department. Ann Emerg Med. 2006 Mar;47(3):237-49. full text*

#22

In the management of acute cardiogenic pulmonary edema with noninvasive ventilation, which of the following were NOT found on meta-analysis?

A. There was a statistically significant decrease in mortality for patients receiving CPAP.

B. There was a statistically significant decrease in mortality for patients receiving noninvasive pressure support ventilation (BIPAP).

C. There was a statistically significant decrease in "need to intubate" for patients receiving CPAP or noninvasive pressure support ventilation (BIPAP).

D. There were no statistically significant differences in mortality when comparing CPAP to noninvasive pressure support ventilation (BIPAP).

E. There was no statistically significant difference in "need to intubate" for patients receiving CPAP versus noninvasive pressure support ventilation (BIPAP).

#22

Answer: B

In the meta-analysis performed by Masip et al., comparing noninvasive ventilation to conventional oxygen therapy in patients with acute pulmonary edema, noninvasive ventilation significantly reduced the mortality rate by nearly 45% compared with conventional therapy (risk ratio [RR], 0.55; 95% CI, 0.40-0.78).

The results were significant for CPAP but not for bilevel ventilation (NIPSV), although there were fewer studies in the NIPSV group. Both modalities showed a significant decrease in the "need to intubate" rate compared with conventional therapy. There were no differences in intubation rates or mortality rates in the analysis of studies comparing the two non-invasive techniques. Noninvasive ventilation should be used in all patients without contraindications who are in significant respiratory distress from pulmonary edema. Although the level of evidence is higher for CPAP, there are no significant differences in clinical outcomes when comparing CPAP vs NIPSV.

- *LLSA 2009: Masip J, et al. Noninvasive ventilation in acute cardiogenic pulmonary edema. Systematic review and meta-analysis. JAMA. 2005; 294: 3124-3130. full text*

#23

In a meta-analysis, which of the following was NOT found to be a sensitive indicator for the diagnosis of cardiac tamponade secondary to a pericardial effusion?

A. Muffled or distant heart sounds

B. Pulsus paradoxus greater than 10 mm

C. Elevated jugular venous pressure

D. Tachycardia

E. Dyspnea

#23

Answer: A

Five features occur in the majority of patients with tamponade. Each has the following sensitivities:

1. Dyspnea (sensitivity range, 87%-89%)
2. Tachycardia (pooled sensitivity, 77%; 95% CI, 69%-85%)
3. Pulsus paradoxus (pooled sensitivity, 82%; 95% CI, 72%-92%)
4. Elevated jugular venous pressure (pooled sensitivity, 76%; 95% CI, 62%-90%)
5. Cardiomegaly on chest radiograph (pooled sensitivity, 89%; 95% CI, 73%-100%)

One study indicated that the presence of pulsus paradoxus greater than 10 mm Hg in a patient with a pericardial effusion increases the likelihood of tamponade (likelihood ratio, 3.3; 95% CI, 1.8-6.3), while a pulsus paradoxus of 10 mm Hg or less greatly lowers the likelihood (likelihood ratio, 0.03; 95% CI, 0.01-0.24).

- *LLSA 2009: Roy CL, et al. Does this patient with a pericardial effusion have cardiac tamponade? JAMA. 2007; 297: 1810-1818. full text*

#24

A patient presents with active chest pain and a 12-lead ECG listed in the choices below. Which of the following according to the ACCF/AHA would NOT meet the criteria for a STEMI?

A. A man with ≥ 1mm ST-segment elevation in lead II, III, and AVF

B. ≥ 1mm ST-segment elevation in lead V4-V6

C. ≥ 2 mm ST segment elevation in V1-V3

D. A woman with 1 mm ST segment elevation in V2 and V3

#24

Answer: D

According to the 2013 ACCF/AHA Guideline for the Management of ST-Elevation Myocardial Infarction and the Universal Definition of Myocardial Infarction, STEMI is defined as new ST elevation at the J point in at least 2 contiguous leads of:

- 2 mm (0.2 mV) in leads V2-V3 (Men)
- 1.5 mm (0.15 mV) in leads V2–V3 (Women)
- 1 mm (0.1mV) in other contiguous chest leads or the limb leads.

There are many alternative causes of ST elevations besides acute infarction. These will be discussed in question 27.

- *ACCF/AHA 2013 ACCF/AHA Guideline for the management of ST-elevation myocardial infarction: a report of the American College of Cardiology Foundation/American Heart Association Task Force on Practice Guidelines. J Am Coll Cardiol. 2013 Jan 29; 61(4):e78-140. full text*

#25

The Sgarbossa criteria can be used to determine the likelihood that a patient with chest pain and a baseline LBBB has a STEMI. Which of the following is NOT a Sgarbossa Criteria?

(Choose two answers.)

A. ST-segment elevation ≥ 1 mm in a lead with an upward QRS complex (5 points)

B. ST-segment depression ≥ 1 mm in V1, V2, V3 (3 points)

C. ST-segment elevation ≥ 5 mm in a lead with downward QRS complex (2 points)

D. ST-segment elevation ≥ 1 mm in a lead with downward QRS complex (2 points)

E. Similar to the general AHA STEMI criteria, the Sgarbossa criteria need to be found in contiguous leads.

#25

Answer: D and E

Unlike the general AHA STEMI criteria, the Sgarbossa criteria need not be found in contiguous leads. In leads with downward QRS complexes, there must be ≥ 5mm ST segment elevation to meet the Sgarbossa criteria.

The criteria are:

1. ST-segment elevation ≥ 1 mm in a lead with an upward QRS complex (5 points)
2. ST-segment depression ≥ 1 mm in V1, V2, V3 (3 points)
3. ST-segment elevation ≥ 5 mm in a lead with downward QRS complex (2 points)

Criterion (1) is more indicative of STEMI than is criterion (2), and the more criteria that are met, the more likely that a STEMI has occurred.

Sgarbossa criteria are poorly sensitive, but highly specific. A score of 5 to 10 indicates an 88 to 100% probability of acute MI. However, with 0 points, there is still a 16% chance of a STEMI.

- *Sgarbossa E, et al. Electrocardiographic diagnosis of evolving acute myocardial infarction in the presence of left bundle-branch block. GUSTO-1 (Global Utilization of Streptokinase and Tissue Plasminogen Activator for Occluded Coronary Arteries) Investigators. NEJM. 1996. 334(8):481-7. full text*

- *Shlipak MG, et al. Should the electrocardiogram be used to guide therapy for patients with left bundle-branch block and suspected myocardial infarction? JAMA. 1999; 281(8): 714. full text*

#26

You are seeing a patient in whom you suspect a patent foramen ovale (PFO). TRUE statements include which of the following?

(Choose three answers.)

A. PFO is the most common type of atrial septal defect.

B. Up to 30% of adults have a PFO.

C. The clinical importance of a PFO lies in its association with paradoxical embolism and stroke.

D. The development of Eisenmenger physiology is accompanied by signs of right ventricular failure and pulmonary hypertension.

#26

Answer: B, C, and D

A PFO may occur in 30% of adults but should not be confused with an atrial septal defect since there is no missing septal tissue Right to left atrial shunting does not generally occur unless the right atrial pressure exceeds the left atrial pressure. Usually the left atrial pressure is greater. However during a valsalva or straining, the right atrial pressure will increase and potentially allow shunting to occur. A PFO can give rise to paradoxical embolization when a venous thrombosis passes across the PFO to the left atria and subsequently enters the arterial circulation. This phenomenon is more likely a complication in children. Eisenmenger syndrome is right ventricular failure due to pulmonary hypertension which leads to further hypoxia. Eisenmenger syndrome in the setting of an isolated PFO without septal defects is rare, due to the low degree of shunted blood.

- *Hara H, et al. Patent foramen ovale: current pathology, pathophysiology, and clinical status. J Am Coll Cardiol. 2005; 46: 1768. full text*

#27

Causes of ST-segment elevation other than ST-segment myocardial infarction include which of the following?

A. Pericarditis

B. Ventricular aneurysm

C. Hyperkalemia

D. Brugada syndrome

E. Hypothermia

F. All of the above

#27

Answer: F

Causes of ST elevation other than acute infarction include:

- Prinzmetal's pattern
- Takotsubo cardiomyopathy
- Post-MI (ventricular aneurysm pattern)
- Acute pericarditis
- Normal "early repolarization variants"
- Left ventricular hypertrophy or left bundle branch block (only V1-V2 or V3)
- Myocarditis (may look like myocardial infarction or pericarditis)
- Brugada patterns (V1-V3 with right bundle branch block-appearing morphology)
- Myocardial tumor
- Myocardial trauma
- Hyperkalemia
- Hypothermia (J wave/Osborn wave)
- Vasospasm (cocaine or sympathomimetic induced)

- *Wang K, et al. ST-segment elevation in conditions other than acute myocardial infarction. N Engl J Med. 2003. Nov 27; 349(22): 2128-35. full text*

#28

Regarding cardiac arrest, which of the following statements is FALSE?

A. The majority of cardiac arrest occur out-of-hospital.

B. Early bystander CPR affects survival outcome.

C. The AHA recommends mouth-to-mouth ventilation interspersed with chest compression for bystander CPR.

D. Bystanders should perform “hands only” CPR and abstain from mouth to mouth.

#28

Answer: C

The vast majority of cardiac arrests occur out of hospital, with survival significantly improved if bystander CPR is initiated. One of the major impediments to bystander CPR was the requirement for mouth-to-mouth ventilation. In 2008 the American Heart Association changed their recommendation to "hands only" or continuous chest compression cardiopulmonary resuscitation (CPR) for untrained lay people. Although Hallstrom, et al. did not find a statistically significant difference, survival to hospital discharge was better among patients who received compression only CPR compared to patients who received compression plus mouth to mouth ventilation.

- *Ramaraj R, et al. Rationale for continuous chest compression cardiopulmonary resuscitation. Heart. 2009 Dec; 95(24): 1978-82.*

- *Hallstrom A, et al. Cardiopulmonary Resuscitation by Chest Compression Alone or with Mouth-to-Mouth Ventilation. N Engl J Med. 2000; 342: 1546-1553. full text*

#29

A 51 year old male is brought into the ED after a cardiac arrest. After chest compressions, defibrillation, and epinephrine, the patient has return of spontaneous circulation (ROSC). He is intubated and unresponsive with intermittent decorticate posturing. You plan to initiate therapeutic hypothermia. TRUE statements about this include which of the following?

(Choose four answers.)

A. If the patient develops an arrhythmia during the cooling process, cooling should be interrupted.

B. For the protocol, the AHA recommends cooling to 32 to 34°C for 12-24 hours.

C. Patients who are comatose prior to cardiac arrest should be excluded from therapeutic hypothermia.

D. Therapeutic hypothermia should not interfere with coronary perfusion, and primary coronary intervention is indicated if the patient has a ST-segment elevation myocardial infarction.

E. Patients should be sedated and paralyzed so that they stop shivering.

#29

Answer: B - E

Cooling should not be interrupted if the patient develops arrhythmias. The AHA currently recommends cooling to 32 to 34 °C for 12 -24 hours for unconscious adult patients with spontaneous circulation after out-of-hospital cardiac arrest when the initial rhythm was ventricular fibrillation or ventricular tachycardia. Targeted temperature management to 36°C may offer the same benefit as traditional cooling to 33°C and should be based on hospital policies. Institutional hypothermia protocols may also encourage cooling of patients with rhythms that were not ventricular fibrillation or ventricular tachycardia.

Sedatives and analgesics should be given to facilitate mechanical ventilation. Intermediate length paralytics such as vecuronium or cisatracurium can decrease shivering, which will allow for greater temperature control and also decrease the patients' stress response and work of breathing. Treatment of suspected underlying acute coronary syndromes with percutaneous coronary intervention or thrombolytics can occur during therapeutic hypothermia, if indicated.

- *Scirica BM. Therapeutic hypothermia after cardiac arrest. Circulation. 2013 Jan 15; 127(2): 244-50. full text*

#30

Regarding the induction of therapeutic hypothermia (TH), which of the following statements is TRUE?

(Choose two answers.)

A. Thrombolytics must not be given during therapeutic hypothermia due to the associated coagulopathy.

B. The patient is most unstable during the rewarming phase (rather than induction or maintenance) of therapeutic hypothermia.

C. When inducing hypothermia, 32-34 °C should be maintained over a 12-24 hour period.

D. The most common rhythm seen with therapeutic hypothermia is sinus bradycardia.

E. When measuring a standard blood gas in a hypothermic patient, the reported pH is overestimated.

#30

Answer: C and D

The most common cardiac rhythm seen with TH is sinus bradycardia. Current AHA guidelines recommend TH with a goal temperature of 32°C to 34°C for 12 to 24 hours in patients successfully resuscitated after cardiac arrest.

Thrombolytics and PCI may be initiated during TH despite the associated coagulopathy. The patient is most unstable during the induction phase, and induction should be performed as rapidly as possible. There may be a mortality increase as high as 20% for every hour delay in cooling.

The blood gas is rewarmed to 37 °C in order to be analyzed. This results in:

- The reported PO_2 being overestimated by 5 mm Hg for every 1°C below 37°C
- The reported PCO_2 being overestimated by 2 mm Hg for every 1°C below 37°C
- The reported pH being underestimated by 0.012 points for every 1°C below 37°C.

- *Polderman KH. Mechanisms of action, physiological effects, and complications of hypothermia. Crit Care Med. 2009 Jul; 37 (7 Suppl): S186-202. full text*
- *Scirica BM. Therapeutic hypothermia after cardiac arrest. Circulation. 2013 Jan 15; 127(2): 244-50. full text*

#31

Regarding myocarditis, which of the following statements is FALSE?

A. Myocarditis may present with a wide range of symptoms, ranging from mild dyspnea or chest pain that resolves without specific therapy to cardiogenic shock and death.

B. The most serious long term complication of myocarditis is dilated cardiomyopathy..

C. Drug-hypersensitivity reactions are the most common cause of myocarditis.

D. Most people with myocarditis who present with acute dilated cardiomyopathy have relatively mild disease that resolves with few short-term sequelae.

#31
Answer: C

Dilated cardiomyopathy with heart failure is the major long-term complication of myocarditis. Infectious etiologies are the most common causes of myocarditis. Other possible causes include autoimmune diseases, medications, and toxins. Reported viral outbreaks of myocarditis include Coxsackievirus B and Parvovirus B19.

Commonly, acute myocarditis may be diagnosed as an unexplained nonischemic dilated cardiomyopathy with worsening symptoms and even decompensation. Other presentations include new onset atrial or ventricular dysrhythmias, heart block, or acute myocardial infarctions. Presenting symptoms are usually non-specific but involve worsening dyspnea, palpitations, chest pain and syncope. Myocarditis also commonly exists with a concomitant pericarditis.

- *LLSA 2011: Cooper LT. Myocarditis. N Engl J Med. 2009 Apr 9; 360(15): 1526-38. full text*

#32

Regarding cocaine induced chest pain, which of the following statements is TRUE?

A. Cocaine was the second most commonly used illicit drug in the United States, second to marijuana, but has now been surpassed by prescription drug abuse.

B. Cocaine causes myocardial ischemia by increasing myocardial oxygen demand, decreasing oxygen supply via vasoconstriction and inducing a prothrombotic state.

C. The presence of chest pain has excellent value for discriminating an ischemic from nonischemic cause in these patients.

D. Ischemia is the only entity that causes chest pain in a cocaine abuser.

#32

Answer: A and B

The most frequent symptom among cocaine users is chest pain. The quality of the pain is often pressure-like but can have a multitude of other qualities. The chest pain alone has little value in determining ischemic vs benign causes in the setting of cocaine use. The pain may also be manifestations of a pneumothorax, arrhythmia, or aortic dissection, caused by the cocaine use. Another less common complication includes an acute pulmonary syndrome called "crack lung". The syndrome involves hypoxemia, hemoptysis, respiratory failure, and diffuse pulmonary infiltrates and occurs after inhalation of freebase cocaine.

Prescription drug abuse is increasing in the United States and has surpassed cocaine use according to the 2012 National Survey on Drug Use and Health, with only marijuana being abused more frequently.

There are four major mechanisms for cocaine induced myocardial ischemia:

- An increase in myocardial oxygen demand from the increased heart rate, blood pressure and contractility
- Decreased cardiac oxygen supply via vasoconstriction and vasospasm
- Induction of a prothrombotic state by stimulating platelet activation and altering the balance between procoagulant and anticoagulant factors
- Accelerated atherosclerosis.

- *LLSA 2011: McCord J, et al. Management of Cocaine-associated chest pain and myocardial infarction. Circulation. 2008; 117: 1897-1907. full text*

- *U.S. Department of Health and Human Services. Results from the 2012 National Survey on Drug Use and Health: Summary of National Findings. full text*

#33

True or False: Cocaine can be detected in the urine 20 days after chronic use on routine urine drug screens.

A. True

B. False

#33

Answer: A

Qualitative detection of the cocaine metabolite benzoylecgonine in the urine is the most commonly used laboratory method for drug screening. Cocaine use is detected as positive when the level of benzoylecgonine is above a standard cut-off value (usually 300 ng/mL). It can be detected in the urine on average from 24 to 48 hours after use. In long-term users, benzoylecgonine has been detected as great as 22 days after last ingestion. This highlights the poor utility of a urine drug screen in the ED for determining if cocaine is causing related chest pain.

- *LLSA 2011. McCord J, et al. Management of Cocaine-associated chest pain and myocardial infarction. Circulation. 2008; 117: 1897-1907. full text*

#34

Regarding cocaine-induced chest pain, which of the following are TRUE?

(Choose two answers.)

A. Unlike patients with ACS unrelated to cocaine use, cocaine users should be provided with intravenous benzodiazepines as early management.

B. Dobutamine echocardiography is contraindicated in a patient who presents with cocaine-induced chest pain.

C. Hypertension and tachycardia should not be the focus of immediate therapy.

D. The ACC/AHA ST-segment–elevation MI guidelines state, "Beta-blockers should be administered to patients with STEMI precipitated by cocaine use."

E. Labetalol has substantial benefits over other beta-blockers in treating cocaine induced hypertension.

#34

Answer: A and C

Treatment of cocaine-chest pain is similar to acute coronary syndrome (ACS) treatment, with only a few modifications. Although there are ACC/AHA recommendations, the evidence is not based on randomized placebo-controlled trials. Early aspirin therapy is recommended since there is greater platelet activation in the setting of cocaine use.

Unlike with ACS, intravenous benzodiazepines (diazepam or lorazepam) relieve chest pain and have beneficial anxiolytic and hemodynamic effects. Treating the underlying anxiety and agitation with a benzodiazepine often decreases the tachycardia and hypertension. However, treatment should not focus on resolution of the hypertension, and should instead be titrated to patient's symptom relief.

If there is a need for emergent correction of hypertension, agents such as sodium nitroprusside, nitroglycerin, or intravenous phentolamine are recommended.

The ACC/AHA ST-segment–elevation MI guidelines state that beta-blockers should be avoided due to the risk of coronary spasm and propranolol is contraindicated. The unopposed alpha adrenergic effects introduced by a beta-blockade has uncertain clinical effects, and the benefits of a mixed alpha and beta blocker, such as labetalol, is theoretical.

Risk stratification in patients with possible ACS or cocaine induced chest pain is still encouraged. There are no contraindications to performing a dobutamine stress test.

- *LLSA 2011. McCord J, et al. Management of Cocaine-associated chest pain and myocardial infarction. Circulation. 2008; 117:1897-1907. full text*

#35

TRUE statements about multifocal atrial tachycardia (MFAT) include which of the following statements?

A. It is a subset of atrial tachycardia.

B. It has more than two foci of impulse formation.

C. On the ECG, at least three distinctly different P waves with varying PR RR, and PP intervals exist.

D. It is often associated with pulmonary disease and hypoxia.

E. All of the above

#35

Answer: E

MFAT is highly associated with pulmonary disease such as COPD. It can also originate from a reentrant focus, and it can be due to electrolyte and acid-base disturbances, drug toxicity, fever, and hypoxia. Note that MFAT often resolves when hypoxia is resolved or with correction of the underlying primary disturbance. MFAT is often confused with atrial fibrillation because both are irregular.

- *Rosen's Emergency Medicine - Concepts and Clinical Practice. 8th edition. 2013. Chapter 79: Dysrhythmias. 1050-1051.*

#36

A 35 year old female with a history of hyperthyroidism on propranolol presents with an intentional overdose of this medication. All of the following are common initial clinical presentations of a propranolol overdose EXCEPT?

A. Bradycardia

B. Bronchospasm and wheezing

C. Hypotension

D. Unconsciousness

#36

Answer: B

Patients with beta-blocker overdoses present most often with profound bradycardia, followed by hypotension and altered mental status. Propranolol is highly lipophilic and causes the most CNS depressant effects of all the beta-blockers. In nonselective and selective beta-blockers, bronchospasm is rarely a complication.

- *Rosen's Emergency Medicine - Concepts and Clinical Practice. 8th edition. 2013. Chapter 152: Cardiovascular Drugs. 1987-1989.*

#37

Regarding left main coronary artery occlusion (LMCO), which of the following statements is TRUE?

A. ≥ 0.5mm ST elevation in lead aVL is consistent with acute LMCO.

B. ≥ 0.5mm ST elevation in lead aVR is consistent with acute LMCO.

C. Acute LMCO is fatal unless there is adequate perfusion from right-sided collaterals.

D. None of the above

E. All of the above

#37

Answer: B

≥ 0.5 mm ST elevation in aVR is consistent with acute LMCO, especially when the degree of ST-elevation in aVR is greater than lead V1, and ST depression is also present in the inferior leads. These ECG findings have >75% sensitivity and specificity for LMCO.

- *LLSA 2013: Rokos IC, et al. Appropriate cardiac cath lab activation: optimizing electrocardiogram interpretation and clinical decision making for acute ST-elevation myocardial infarction. Am Heart J. 2010; 160: 995-1003. full text*

#38

Regarding treatment of patients resuscitated from sudden cardiac arrest, which of the following statements is TRUE?

A. The number needed to treat (NNT) with therapeutic hypothermia to improve rate of cerebral recovery is approximately 100.

B. The target hypothermia temperature is 37°C.

C. Baseline abnormal neurologic status immediately after ROSC precludes early cath lab activation

D. The patient should be cooled for 72 hours.

E. The patient should be rewarmed over 8 hours after the initial 24hr cooling.

#38

Answer: E

The NNT is approximately 6 for therapeutic hypothermia. Neurologic status after return of spontaneous circulation (ROSC) should not determine the need for cardiac catheterization. Prognostication on neurologic outcome should not occur until at least 72 hours after rewarming. Although the best hypothermia protocol has yet to be definitively proven, current evidence suggests two potentially equivalent options. Cooling as early as possible (pre-arrival to cath lab) to a target temperature of:

- 33 °C and maintenance of 33 degrees for 24 hours
- 36 °C and maintenance of 36 degrees for 24 hours

After 24 hours of cooling, the patient should then be rewarmed over 8 hours (0.5 degrees per hour) back to normothermia.

- *TheNNT.com - Mild Therapeutic Hypothermia for Neuroprotection Following Cardiopulmonary Resuscitation (CPR). http://www.thennt.com/nnt/hypothermia-for-neuroprotection-after-cardiac-arrest/*

- *Nielsen N, et al. Targeted Temperature Management at 33°C versus 36°C after Cardiac Arrest. N Engl J Med. 2013. 369(23): 2197-2206. full text*

#39

A patient with long-standing CHF, taking amiodarone presents to the ED due to ICD firing. Interrogation of his ICD shows that he had an episode of ventricular fibrillation for 15 seconds when the firing occurred. What should be done with this patient?

A. No need for any evaluation since this was an appropriate shock

B. If the device fires repeatedly in the ED in the absence of a detectable dysrhythmia, then a bolus of amiodarone is indicated.

C. Admit the patient for monitoring

#39

Answer: C

Ideally, these patients should be seen in the ED by cardiology. Almost all patients with a shockable event should be admitted for monitoring and observation. Although the ICD acted appropriately, titration of medications may be needed. Deactivation of an inappropriately firing ICD can occur in the ED, but the patient should have cardiac resuscitation equipment at bedside in case of a future dysrhythmia. Amiodarone will not affect an inappropriately firing ICD.

- *Roberts and Hedges' Clinical Procedures in Emergency Medicine. 6th edition. 2013. Chapter: 13 Assessment of Implantable Devices. 248-262.*

#40

You are seeing a patient who presents with chest pain and shortness of breath. The chest X-ray demonstrates air in the pericardial space. Possible risk factors for a pneumopericardium include which of the following?

A. Esophageal diverticulum

B. Asthma

C. Barotrauma from positive-pressure ventilation

D. Cocaine inhalation from a positive pressure device

E. All of the above

#40

Answer: E

Pneumopericardium is caused by a connection between the pericardium and the pleural, bronchi, or GI tract. Gas producing bacteria can also cause the phenomenon. Fistulization with the GI tract can occur from GI malignancy (specifically esophagus or stomach), peptic ulcer disease, or esophageal diverticula. Barotrauma, asthma, rapid increase in intrathoracic pressure (Valsalva) and drug inhalation can also cause pneumopericardium.

- *Rosen's Emergency Medicine - Concepts and Clinical Practice. 8th edition. 2013. Chapter 82: Pericardial and Myocardial Disease.1097-1098.*

#41

Pacemaker malfunction can be separated into broad categories:

- **Failure to capture**
- **Undersensing**
- **Oversensing**
- **Inappropriate rate**

True or False: Battery depletion can lead to all of these problems.

A. True

B. False

#41

Answer: B

Battery depletion can lead to failure to capture and an inappropriate rate. Causes of undersensing can be due to lead displacement, inadequate endocardial lead contact, low-voltage intracardiac P-waves or QRS complexes, and lead fracture. Oversensing is due to sensing extracardiac signals and T wave sensing.

- *Rosen's Emergency Medicine - Concepts and Clinical Practice. 8th edition. 2013. Chapter 80: Implantable Cardiac Devices. 1068-1071.*

#42

TRUE statements about post-cardiac arrest management include which of the following?

(Choose two answers.)

A. Arterial hyperoxia (PaO2 >300 mm Hg) may be beneficial.

B. Hypoxia should be avoided.

C. Hypocarbia should be avoided.

D. Hyperventilation should be initiated.

#42

Answer: B and C

Hyperoxia is independently associated with increased in-hospital mortality. Often 100% oxygen is used for resuscitation but should be rapidly titrated down to the minimum needed for an arterial saturation of 94%. Hyperventilation should be avoided because it produces hypocarbia, causing cerebral vasoconstriction and decreased cerebral perfusion. Additionally, hyperventilation can cause auto-PEEP and decrease cardiac output.

- *Stub D, et al. Post Cardiac arrest syndrome. A review of therapeutic strategies. Circulation. 2011; 12: 1428-1435. full text*

#43

Regarding therapeutic hypothermia (TH) in the post-ROSC management, which of the following is TRUE?

A. Of all cooling mechanisms, the General Electric device has been demonstrated to be the most effective.

B. Possible adverse effects of TH include electrolyte imbalances and altered coagulation profile.

C. TH increases the heart rate and decreases the systemic vascular resistance.

D. Prehospital induction of TH has been found to be more beneficial when compared with cooling patients on arrival to the hospital.

#43

Answer: B

There has not been a demonstrated benefit from using one particular cooling device over any other device in regard to mortality or morbidity. Prehospital cooling has also not been shown to offer a clinical mortality benefit when compared to in-hospital cooling. TH decreases heart rate, and bradycardia is the most common dysrhythmia. There is also an increase in systemic vascular resistance. Hypothermia can cause electrolyte changes, diuresis, hypovolemia, and coagulopathies.

- *Stub D, et al. Post Cardiac arrest syndrome. A review of therapeutic strategies. Circulation. 2011; 12: 1428-1435. full text*

#44

Which of the following is a predictor of poor prognosis after cardiac arrest.

A. Patient comorbidities

B. Arrest details, such as initial rhythm, time to ROSC, absence of bystander CPR, and maximal end-tidal CO2

C. Both of the above

D. Neither of the above

#44

Answer: C

All the above factors are associated with patient outcome but none can definitively predict if care should be withdrawn. Absent pupillary and corneal reflexes at day 3 after rewarming are predictors of very poor prognosis. Neurologic prognostication should be delayed until 3 days after rewarming.

- *Stub D, et al. Post Cardiac arrest syndrome. A review of therapeutic strategies. Circulation. 2011; 12: 1428-1435. full text*

#45

Hospital-based strategies to decrease time to treatment in primary percutaneous coronary intervention should include all of the following EXCEPT:

A. "Facilitated PCI" – transferring patients to a hospital capable of PCI after a half dose or full dose of a thrombolytic is administered

B. Prehospital ECG and activation

C. ED activation of the catheterization laboratory

D. Establishment of the expectation that the PCI team can arrive within 20-30 minutes of activation

E. Routine data monitoring with prompt feedback

#45

Answer: A

Attempts are always ongoing to improve door to balloon time. A strategy named "Facilitated PCI" referred to treatment with a fibrinolytic and a glycoprotein IIb/IIIa receptor blockers followed by PCI.

However, clinical trials were not able to demonstrate improved patient centered outcomes with facilitated PCI. In fact, there may actually be increased mortality. For rural areas and long transport times, there may be local protocols for facilitated PCI, but it is not a widespread recommendation. There may in fact be harm, if a full-dose fibrinolytic is administered prior to transfer.

- *Nallamothu BK, et al. Time to treatment in primary percutaneous coronary intervention. N Engl J Med. 2007; 357: 1631-1648. full text*

#46

Regarding myocarditis, which of the following statements is TRUE?

(Choose three answers.)

A. The sensitivity of the electrocardiogram for myocarditis is high and there are always associated signs of pericarditis.

B. Cardiac MRI is being used with increasing frequency as a diagnostic test in suspected acute myocarditis.

C. All patients with suspected myocarditis should undergo an endomyocardial biopsy, since this is the gold standard for diagnosis.

D. The mainstay of therapy for acute myocarditis is supportive therapy for left ventricular dysfunction.

E. In patients with acute myocarditis, therapy for arrhythmias is also supportive, since arrhythmias usually resolve after the acute phase of the disease.

#46

Answer: B, D, and E

In acute myocarditis, patients most often have ECGs with sinus tachycardia and nonspecific ST-segment and T-wave abnormalities. Patients can often be misdiagnosed with a STEMI. Since myocarditis and pericarditis frequently coexist, ECG findings consistent with pericarditis, such as PR depression, may also be present. Overall, the sensitivity of the electrocardiogram for myocarditis is low (47%).

Treatment of heart failure should follow standard care, with preload and afterload reduction and optimization of contractility. Supportive care is also employed for new onset arrhythmias but may require cardioverter-defibrillator implantation.

Endomyocardial biopsy may be an option in patients in whom the etiology of the myocarditis from other infiltrative diseases such as amyloidosis must be made. However, cardiac MRI is used more often as a non-invasive diagnostic modality.

- *LLSA 2011: Cooper LT. Myocarditis. N Engl J Med. 2009 Apr 9; 360(15): 1526-38. full text*

CRITICAL CARE

#1

Regarding propofol administration for conscious sedation, which of the following is FALSE?

A. An absolute contraindication to its use is an allergy to egg or soy-based products.

B. One known adverse side effect is hypotension.

C. It is an analgesic.

D. It is a sedative.

E. It causes amnesia.

#1

Answer: C

Propofol is a sedative amnestic without analgesic properties. The amnesia lasts an average of 15 minutes in adults who have received 1 mg/kg of propofol followed by 0.5 mg/kg until sedated. Onset of sedation is approximately 30 seconds after the initial bolus. The major side effect of propofol is hypotension, as well as apnea. The hypotensive effects are more profound in patients with depleted intravascular volumes.

- *LLSA 2009: Miner JR, Burton JH. Clinical Practice Advisory: Emergency department procedural sedation with propofol. Ann Emerg Med. 2007; 50: 182-187. full text*

#2

In patients with septic shock, hydrocortisone appears to:

A. Improve survival in all patients with septic shock

B. Improve survival in patients who do not have a response to corticotropin

C. Hasten reversal of shock in patients in whom shock was reversed

D. Decrease the recurrence of sepsis and septic shock and fewer episodes of superinfection

E. Improve patient survival in those with hemorrhagic shock

#2

Answer: C

Hydrocortisone is widely used in patients with septic shock even though a survival benefit has only been reported in patients remaining hypotensive after fluid and vasopressor resuscitation and whose plasma cortisol levels did not rise appropriately after the administration of corticotropin.

In the the multicenter, randomized, double-blind, placebo-controlled CORTICUS trial by Sprung et al, 251 patients received 50 mg of intravenous hydrocortisone and 248 patients received placebo every 6 hours for 5 days; the dose was then tapered during a 6-day period.

The primary outcome was death at 28 days in patients who did not have a response to a corticotropin test. Of the 499 patients in the study, 233 (46.7%) did not have a response to corticotropin (125 in the hydrocortisone group and 108 in the placebo group). At 28 days, there was no significant difference in mortality between patients in the two study groups who did not have a response to corticotropin (39.2% in the hydrocortisone group and 36.1% in the placebo group, P=0.69) or between those who had a response to corticotropin (28.8% in the hydrocortisone group and 28.7% in the placebo group).

Death at 28 days occurred in 86 patients from the hydrocortisone group (34.3%) and 78 in the placebo group (31.5%).

However, shock was reversed more quickly than in the placebo group but at the expense of a greater number of superinfections that resulted in new sepsis. There was no improvement in overall survival with patients who received hydrocortisone, although in those who had recovery from shock, hydrocortisone increased the speed of recovery.

- *Sprung CL, et al. Hydrocortisone therapy for patients with septic shock. N Engl J Med. 2008; 358: 111-124. full text*

#3

Which of the following patients will desaturate to less than 90% oxygen saturation most quickly during rapid sequence intubation without pre-oxygenation?

A. Healthy young adult

B. Morbidly obese pregnant female at 39 weeks gestation

C. Pregnant female at 39 weeks gestation

D. Normal, healthy infant

E. Normal, healthy child

#3

Answer: B

Any patient who may require endotracheal intubation should be given adequate preoxygenation to allow for "nitrogen washout" of the lungs. A healthy 70 kg adult can maintain oxygen saturation above 90% for eight minutes. Young children typically fall below the 90% threshold in less than four minutes. The oxygen saturation of adults with severe illness or obesity and pregnant women nearing the end of their third trimester, fall below 90% in less than three minutes.

Preoxygenation provides a longer period before clinically significant desaturation occurs, regardless of the patient's condition. Although the duration of time before desaturation varies significantly, "nitrogen washout" can be achieved with the patient taking eight vital capacity (ie, maximal) breaths. Passive oxygenation with nasal cannula during the procedure may also increase the time period before desaturation occurs.

- *Rosen's Emergency Medicine - Concepts and Clinical Practice. 8th edition. 2013. Chapter 1: Airway. 13-14.*

#4

You decide to use succinylcholine to intubate a patient. True statements about succinylcholine include all of the following, EXCEPT:

A. It is contraindicated in a patient who sustained a 40% TBSA burn 30 minutes prior to arrival.

B. Onset of action is 45 to 60 seconds.

C. Duration of action is 6-10 minutes.

D. It may be administered intramuscularly, but when given via that route, the dose should be doubled.

E. The dose is 1.5 – 2 mg/kg IV.

#4

Answer: A

Succinylcholine is a neuromuscular blocking agent (1.5-2 mg/kg IV or 3-4 mg/kg IM), that acts by directly depolarizing the neuromuscular junction. It has a rapid rate of onset for paralysis (45 to 60 seconds) and brief duration of action (6 to 10 minutes). Since succinylcholine is a depolarizing agent, in conditions where there is upregulation of receptors in the neuromuscular junction, there can be transient increases in potassium, causing hyperkalemia. Thus, succinylcholine should be avoided in patients with established conditions (longer than 5 days) that cause upregulation of receptors at the neuromuscular junction, for example:

- Spinal cord injury
- Stroke
- Denervating disease such as multiple sclerosis
- Major burns
- Myopathy
- Rhabdomyolysis
- History of malignant hyperthermia

- Rosen's Emergency Medicine - Concepts and Clinical Practice. 8th edition. 2013. Chapter 1: Airway. 13-14.

#5

Regarding the use of hydrocortisone in septic shock patients, which of the following was found

A. Mortality was significantly reduced in patients who received steroids.

B. Mortality was only reduced in patients who had a positive corticotropin test.

C. Mortality was only reduced in patients who had a negative corticotropin test.

D. Shock was reversed more quickly in the steroid group, when compared to the placebo group.

E. There were fewer episodes of superinfection in the steroid group.

#5

Answer: D

In summary, the use of hydrocortisone did not decrease mortality in a general population of patients with septic shock, even though the drug hastened reversal of shock. This lack of improvement may be related to an increased incidence of superinfection and new septic episodes. No benefit was seen in a subgroup of patients who had had no response to corticotropin, as was shown previously for patients with severe septic shock. This finding may be related to methodologic issues surrounding the accurate diagnosis of adrenal insufficiency in critically ill patients or to decreased prognostic importance of this phenomenon in less severe shock. On the basis of these findings, hydrocortisone is not recommended as general adjuvant therapy for septic shock that is fluid or vasopressor-responsive. Corticotropin testing is also not recommended for determining which patients should receive hydrocortisone therapy. At the expense of increasing the risk for infection, hydrocortisone may have a role among patients who are treated early after the onset of septic shock who remain hypotensive despite the administration of high-dose vasopressors.

- *LLSA 2010: Sprung CL, et al. Hydrocortisone therapy for patients with septic shock. N Engl J Med. 2008; 358: 111-124. full text*

#6

You are just about to intubate someone, and you are considering the use of succinylcholine. Consider using a nondepolarizing agent in which of the following conditions?

A. Personal history of malignant hyperthermia

B. Burn over 72 hours

C. Rhabdomyolysis

D. Stroke greater than 72 hours

E. Hyperkalemia

F. All of the above

#6

Answer: F

A nondepolarizing neuromuscular blocking agent should be considered when performing RSI on patients with the following conditions:

1. Malignant hyperthermia history (personal or familial)
2. Neuromuscular disease
3. Muscular dystrophy
4. Stroke over 72 hours old
5. Rhabdomyolysis
6. Burn over 72 hours old
7. Significant hyperkalemia (eg, suggested by characteristic changes on an electrocardiogram).

- *Rosen's Emergency Medicine - Concepts and Clinical Practice. 8th edition. 2013. Chapter 1: Airway. 13-14.*

#7

Noninvasive ventilation (NIV) is a modality of ventilatory support without endotracheal intubation and sedation that has demonstrated to be useful in several forms of respiratory failure. Regarding NIV for the treatment of cardiogenic pulmonary edema, which of the following statements is FALSE?

A. Continuous positive airway pressure (CPAP) may be performed with an oxygen source connected to a tight-fitting face mask with an expiratory valve to maintain constant positive pressure.

B. Bilevel noninvasive pressure support ventilation (NIPSV) is more complex, requires a ventilator to provide 2 levels of pressure: one to assist patients with inspiratory positive airway pressure (IPAP) and the other, like CPAP, to maintain expiratory positive pressure (EPAP).

C. A quantitative systematic review of existing literature demonstrated that NIV reduces intubation rate and mortality in patients with acute pulmonary edema.

D. NIPSV is clearly superior to CPAP in terms of its impact on mortality and intubation rates for pulmonary edema.

E. Noninvasive ventilation has recently been categorized as class IIa, level of evidence A, in the guidelines on the diagnosis and treatment for acute heart failure by the European Society of Cardiology.

#7

Answer: D

Masip et al. performed a systematic review and quantitative analysis of the short-term effect of noninvasive ventilation on major clinical outcomes in acute cardiogenic pulmonary edema. They selected fifteen trials. Overall, noninvasive ventilation significantly reduced the mortality rate by nearly 45% compared with conventional therapy (risk ratio [RR], 0.55; 95% [CI], 0.40-0.78).

The results were significant for CPAP (RR, 0.53; 95% CI, 0.35-0.81) but not for noninvasive pressure support ventilation (NIPSV) (RR, 0.60; 95% CI, 0.34-1.05), although there were fewer studies in the latter.

Both modalities showed a significant decrease in the "need to intubate" rate compared with conventional therapy: CPAP (RR, 0.40; 95% CI, 0.27-0.58), NIPSV (RR, 0.48; 95% CI, 0.30-0.76), and together (RR, 0.43; 95% CI, 0.32-0.57).

There were no differences in intubation or mortality rates in the analysis of studies comparing the 2 techniques.

- *LLSA 2009: Masip J, et al. Noninvasive ventilation in acute cardiogenic pulmonary edema. JAMA. 2005; 294:3124-3130. full text*

#8

True or False: The available evidence suggests that etomidate suppresses adrenal function.

A. True

B. False

#8

Answer: A

True. According to this systematic review of 20 studies, pooled mean cortisol levels were lower in elective surgical patients induced with etomidate compared with those induced with other agents between 1 and 4 hours post induction. However, none of the studies showed a statistically significant effect on mortality, and no studies to date have been powered to detect a difference in hospital, ventilator, or ICU length of stay.

- *LLSA 2010: Hohl CM, et al. The effect of a bolus dose of etomidate on cortisol levels, mortality, and health services utilization: a systematic review. Ann Emerg Med. 2010; 56: 105-113.*

#9

You are treating a patient with septic shock, and after performing aggressive fluid resuscitation, consider escalating to vasopressor therapy. You are debating between dopamine vs. norepinephrine to restore and maintain blood pressure. Regarding these two vasopressors in the treatment of shock, which of the following is FALSE?

A. Both of these agents influence alpha-adrenergic and beta-adrenergic receptors, but to different degrees.

B. There is no significant difference between the two vasopressors in rate of all-cause death at 29 days, 6 months, or 12 months.

C. Patients who are treated with norepinephrine are more likely to have an arrhythmia.

D. Patients with cardiogenic shock have a higher rate of death if treated with dopamine when compared to those who are treated with norepinephrine.

E. Dopamine is a less potent vasopressor than norepinephrine.

#9

Answer: C

In a multicenter, randomized trial, performed by De-Backer et al., patients with shock were randomized to receive either dopamine or norepinephrine. The primary outcome variable was death. The trial included 1679 patients, and there was no significant between-group difference in mortality at 28 days (52.5% in the dopamine group and 48.5% in the norepinephrine group; odds ratio with dopamine, 1.17; 95% confidence interval, 0.97 to 1.42; P=0.10). However, there were more arrhythmic events among the patients treated with dopamine than among those treated with norepinephrine (207 events [24.1%] vs. 102 events [12.4%], P<0.001).

A subgroup analysis showed that dopamine, as compared with norepinephrine, was associated with a higher mortality among the 280 patients with cardiogenic shock but not among the 1044 patients with septic shock or the 263 with hypovolemic shock.

- *LLSA 2012: DeBacker D, et al. Comparison of dopamine and norepinephrine in the treatment of shock. N Engl J Med. 2010; 362: 779-789. full text*

#10

You are about to perform rapid sequence intubation, and you ask the nurse to order up etomidate. The medical student who is "shadowing" you asks if etomidate increases mortality. You state that:

(Choose two answers.)

A. Etomidate inhibits cortisol production by blocking 11-beta hydroxylase but has not been shown to affect mortality.

B. Etomidate is the most widely used induction agent in North America and appears safe even though it does transiently suppress adrenal function.

C. A review of the literature demonstrated an overwhelming effect on increasing hospital length of stay when etomidate was used for induction.

D. Multiple studies have shown a significant effect on increased ventilator days when etomidate was used for induction.

E. A review of the literature showed a statistically significant difference in mortality, favoring the use of etomidate.

#10

Answer: A and B

In a systematic review by Hohl CM et al., pooled mean cortisol levels were lower in elective surgical patients induced with etomidate compared with those induced with other agents between 1 and 4 hours post induction. The differences varied from 6.1 microg/dL (95% CI, 2.4 to 9.9 microg/dL) to 16.4 microg/dL (95% CI, 9.7 to 23.1 microg/dL).

Two studies in critically ill patients reported significantly different cortisol levels up to 7 hours post induction. None of the studies demonstrated (pooled estimate odds ratio 1.14; 95% CI 0.81 to 1.60) a statistically significant effect on mortality. Only one study reported longer ventilator, ICU, and hospital lengths of stay in patients intubated with etomidate. The available evidence suggests that etomidate suppresses adrenal function transiently without demonstrating a significant effect on mortality. However, no studies to date have been powered to detect a difference in hospital, ventilator, or ICU length of stay or in mortality.

- *LLSA 2012: Hohl CM, et al. The effect of a bolus dose of etomidate on cortisol levels, mortality, and health services utilization: a systematic review. Ann Emerg Med. 2010; 56: 105-113. full text*

#11

In a study comparing etomidate and ketamine for RSI in acutely ill patients, which of the following was TRUE?

A. Ketamine led to greater difficulty in intubation.

B. Etomidate led to higher 28 day mortality.

C. Ketamine led to longer duration of catecholamine weaning.

D. Length of stay was longer with etomidate.

E. None of the above

#11

Answer: E

In a randomized, controlled, single-blind trial by Jabre et al, 655 patients who needed sedation for emergency intubation were prospectively enrolled from 12 emergency medical services or emergency departments and 65 intensive care units in France. Patients were randomly assigned to receive 0.3 mg/kg of etomidate (n=328) or 2 mg/kg of ketamine (n=327) for intubation. The primary endpoint was the maximum score of the sequential organ failure assessment (SOFA) during the first 3 days in the intensive care unit. The mean maximum SOFA score between the two groups did not differ significantly (10.3 [SD 3.7] for etomidate vs 9.6 [3.9] for ketamine; mean difference 0.7 [95% CI 0.0-1.4], p=0.056). Intubation conditions did not differ significantly between the two groups (median intubation difficulty score 1 [IQR 0-3] in both groups; p=0.70). The percentage of patients with adrenal insufficiency was significantly higher in the etomidate group than in the ketamine group (OR 6.7, 3.5-12.7). There were no serious adverse events with either study drug, and there were no differences in mortality, duration of catecholamine weaning, or length of stay.

- *LLSA 2012: Jabre P, et al. Etomidate versus Ketamine for rapid sequence intubation in acutely ill patients: a multicentre randomized controlled trial. Lancet. 2009; 374: 293-300. full text*

#12

You are about to intubate a morbidly obese patient. TRUE statements about managing the airway in obese patients include which of the following statements?

A. Obese patients have lower pH of gastric contents.

B. Obese patients have greater total lung capacity and vital capacity.

C. Airway resistance is decreased in obesity.

D. Etomidate should be dosed according to lean body mass.

E. Ketamine should be dosed according to total body weight.

#12

Answer: A

Obese patients have a higher incidence of GERD and have lower gastric pH, which puts them at risk for lung injury after aspiration. Obese patients may undergo oxygen desaturation to 90% within 3 minutes compared to 6 minutes in normal weight patients. In patients with BMI greater than 60, the time to desaturation may be less than one minute. Obesity causes diminished total lung capacity and vital capacity from decreased chest wall compliance and increased abdominal cavity contents. Airway resistance is also increased in obesity, and they have a higher incidence of hypoxemia and hypercapnia. Etomidate is lipophilic and theoretically should be administered according to total body weight. Ketamine should be dosed according to lean body mass, by adding 20% to the ideal body weight.

- *LLSA 2012: Dagin J, Medson R. Emergency department management of the airway in obese adults. Ann Emerg Med. 2010;56:95-104.*

#13

TRUE statements about airway management in the obese patient include:

(Choose three answers.)

A. Noninvasive positive pressure ventilation is not well-tolerated by the obese.

B. The patient's head should be elevated 25 degrees (ramped position).

C. Succinylcholine should be administered based upon total body weight.

D. Rocuronium should be administered based upon total body weight.

E. Video laryngoscopy has been shown to improve visualization of the larynx and reduce the time to tracheal intubation in obese patients undergoing elective surgery.

#13

Answer: B, C, and E

In the morbidly obese patient, the head and shoulders should be elevated above the chest such that the external auditory canal is parallel with the sternal notch to optimize the laryngoscopic view.

Multiple folded blankets placed under the head, shoulders, and neck may be required to achieve the so-called ramped position. Application of 100% oxygen with pressure support before tracheal intubation increases the duration of non-hypoxic apnea by 1 minute in obese patients undergoing elective surgery (decreases atelectasis and increases functional residual capacity).

When succinylcholine is administered according to ideal body weight, poorer laryngoscopic views and incomplete neuromuscular paralysis are achieved compared with dosing based on total body weight. Inadequate sedation and muscle relaxation may predispose to aspiration. Succinylcholine should be dosed according to TOTAL body weight. Nondepolarizing neuromuscular agents, such as rocuronium should be dosed according to IDEAL body weight.

- *LLSA 2012: Dagin J, Medson R. Emergency department management of the airway in obese adults. Ann Emerg Med. 2010; 56: 95-104.*

- *Meyhoff CS, et al. Should dosing of rocuronium in obese patients be based on ideal or corrected body weight? Anesth Analg. 2009 Sep; 109(3): 787-92*

- *Airway Cam - Ear Sternal Notch http://www.airwaycam.com/Ear-Sternal-Notch-Positioning.html*

#14.

When comparing etomidate versus ketamine for rapid sequence intubation in acutely ill patients, which of the following statements is TRUE?

A. Etomidate is the sedative-hypnotic drug that is used most frequently in rapid sequence intubation.

B. A single bolus of etomidate is associated with a significant increase in morbidity and mortality compared with ketamine in patients admitted to the intensive care unit.

C. Etomidate affects the adrenal axis, and according to one study, more than 4/5 of etomidate recipients had adrenal insufficiency and were non-responders to the ACTH stimulation test.

D. No patients given ketamine in an RCT of ketamine versus etomidate developed adrenal insufficiency.

E. Serious adverse events are more common in the etomidate group.

#14

Answer: A and C

According to a randomized controlled trial by Jabre et al. with 655 patients, the percentage of patients with adrenal insufficiency was significantly higher in the etomidate group than in the ketamine group (OR 6.5, 95%CI 3.5-12.7), but there were no serious adverse events with either study drug. Statement C is true, and **about half of patients given ketamine also had adrenal insufficiency**. This emphasizes that critical illness per se affects adrenal function. These authors emphasize that ketamine is a safe and valuable alternative to etomidate for endotracheal intubation in critically ill patients, and should be considered in those with sepsis.

- *LLSA 2012: Jabre P, et al. Etomidate versus ketamine for rapid sequence intubation in acutely ill patients: a multicentre randomized controlled trial. Lancet. 2009;374:293-300.*

#15

With respect to proper positioning of the morbidly obese patient for laryngoscopy and intubation, which of the following statements is TRUE?

A. The head and shoulders should be made parallel to the chest.

B. The head and shoulders should be lower than the chest.

C. The "sniffing" position is the optimal position.

D. The head and shoulders should be elevated above the chest.

E. None of the above

#15

Answer: D

Repositioning the morbidly obese patient after failed attempts can be difficult and time consuming, and proper positioning should be achieved before any attempts at laryngoscopy. In the morbidly obese patient, the head and shoulders should be elevated above the chest such that the external auditory canal is parallel with the sternal notch to optimize view during laryngoscopy. Multiple folded blankets placed under the head, shoulders, and neck may be required to achieve the so-called ramped position, which improves laryngoscopic view over the standard “sniffing” position in obese patients. The ramped position may also improve mask ventilation and provide easy access to the neck for application of cricoid pressure and attempts at a surgical airway.

- *LLSA 2012: Dargin J and Medzon R. Emergency Department Management of the airway in obese adults. Ann Emerg Med. 2010; 56: 95-104.*
- *Airway Cam - Ear Sternal Notch http://www.airwaycam.com/Ear-Sternal-Notch-Positioning.html*

#16

When confirming endotracheal intubation in the morbidly obese patient, which of the following statements is TRUE?

A. Pulse oximetry may be inaccurate because of poor light-wave transmission through increased soft tissue in the fingers.

B. Condensation in the endotracheal may be less effective in morbidly obese patients.

C. Interpretation of chest radiography can prove challenging as well, owing to poor penetration of radiographs through excess soft tissue.

D. All of the above

E. None of the above

#16

Answer: D

All of the statements are true. Reliance on indirect clinical tests alone, such as chest and gastric auscultation, chest excursions, endotracheal tube condensation, and oxygen saturations to detect esophageal tracheal intubation contributes to hypoxemia, regurgitation, aspiration, and cardiovascular complications during emergency airway management. Obesity may further diminish the utility of clinical findings to confirm endotracheal tube placement. End tidal CO_2 detection should be used in all intubated patients.

- *LLSA 2012: Dargin J and Medzon R. Emergency Department Management of the airway in obese adults. Ann Emerg Med. 2010; 56: 95-104.*

#17

When comparing dopamine versus norepinephrine in the treatment of shock, which of the following statements is TRUE?

A. In a multicenter RCT comparing dopamine vs. norepinephrine as the initial vasopressor in the treatment of shock, there was a significant benefit of norepinephrine in the rate of death at 28 days.

B. Dopamine was associated with more arrhythmic events.

C. In a subgroup analysis of patients with septic shock, patients in this particular group had a lower mortality when treated with norepinephrine.

D. None of the above

E. All of the above

#17

Answer: B

Although there was no significant difference in the rate of death between patients with shock who were treated with dopamine as the first-line vasopressor agent and those who were treated with norepinephrine, the use of dopamine was associated with more arrhythmic events, and these events were severe enough to require withdrawal from the study. In addition, dopamine was associated with a significant increase in the rate of death in the predefined subgroup of patients with cardiogenic shock, even though one might expect cardiac output to be better maintained with dopamine than with norepinephrine.

- *DeBacker D, et al. Comparison of dopamine and norepinephrine in the treatment of shock. N Engl J Med. 2010; 362(9): 779-789. full text*

#18

True or False: In severe obstructive airway disease, the inspiratory to expiratory ratio (I:E) should be about 1:1.

A. True

B. False

#18

Answer: B

Exhalation times must be prolonged or dangerous breath-stacking occurs. I:E ratios should be 1:5 or less to promote full exhalation. Because respiratory frequency is the single greatest determinant of expiratory time, tachypnea is the greatest enemy of asthmatics on positive pressure ventilation.

- *LLSA 2013: Manthous CA. Avoiding circulatory complications during endotracheal intubation and initiation of positive pressure ventilation. J Emerg Med. 2010; 38(5): 622-31. full text*

#19

According to the landmark ARDSnet study, which of the following strategies is indicated to prevent worsening lung injury?

A. Tidal volumes of 10 ml/kg.

B. Plateau pressure to be maintained at >45 cm

C. Increase PEEP to achieve >90% oxygen saturation

D. Maintain patient-ventilator synchrony

#19

Answer: C and D

Tidal volumes should be 6 ml/kg. The plateau pressure should be checked and maintained less than 30 cm H_2O Hg. Tidal volumes may need to be decreased to ensure safe plateau pressures. Patient-ventilator synchrony should be maintained because positive end expiratory pressure (PEEP) is less useful in settings of over-breathing, coughing, and ventilator dyssynchrony.

- *LLSA 2013: Manthous CA. Avoiding circulatory complications during endotracheal intubation and initiation of positive pressure ventilation. J Emerg Med. 2010; 38(5): 622-31. full text*

#20

You have just intubated a patient with severe asthma.

True or False: A higher peak airway pressure may be tolerated as long as tidal volumes are titrated to yield a plateau pressure < 30 cm H_2O.

A. True

B. False

#20

Answer: A

Hypoventilation is a risk of severe obstruction because ventilators are often programmed to stop tidal volume deliveries after exceeding a certain peak airway pressure (commonly 40-60 cm H_2O). In severe asthma, when peak airway pressure reflects resistance of the upper airways, the ventilator may truncate breaths to dangerously low volumes, barely sufficient to ventilate the dead space. So, the allowable peak airway pressures must be set higher, so long as plateau pressure is maintained < 30 cm H_2O.

- *LLSA 2013: Manthous CA. Avoiding circulatory complications during endotracheal intubation and initiation of positive pressure ventilation. J Emerg Med. 2010; 38(5): 622-31. full text*

#21

True or False: National guidelines suggest no more than three ETI attempts before either inviting more skilled personnel or employing "difficult airway" adjuncts.

A. True

B. False

#21

Answer: A

True. Note that BVM should only be interrupted for at most, 30 seconds and the maximum oxygen saturation should be achieved prior to each attempt. Vital signs should be monitored carefully for bradycardia, excessive tachycardia, hypotension and desaturation, which should prompt return to BVM even if 30 seconds has not elapsed.

- *LLSA 2013: Manthous CA. Avoiding circulatory complications during endotracheal intubation and initiation of positive pressure ventilation. J Emerg Med. 2010; 38(5): 622-31. full text*

#22

More than 25% of patients develop transient hypotension after emergent ETI and positive pressure ventilation. Some of the ways in which this can be avoided include which of the following?

A. Begin volume resuscitation – in all but obviously hypervolemic patients during ETI, especially when patients are very catecholamine driven before ETI.

B. Ensure that a pure vasoconstrictor, such as phenylephrine, is rapidly available, in case fluid resuscitation is insufficient to fill the vascular system until the patient awakes.

C. Ventilate with tidal volumes of 6-8 mL/kg of ideal body weight.

D. All of the above

#22

Answer: D

One other consideration would be to attempt ETI with intermittent doses rather than bolus doses of sedatives. For example 1-2 mg of midazolam or lorazepam or 0.3 mg/kg of propofol every 5-10 minutes if the patient's clinical status allows. Other agents such as ketamine provide an adjunctive catecholamine release for further hemodynamic stability. Using small incremental doses will prevent overdosing that could potentially induce hypotension. Also beginning with fairly low ventilator settings will allow for titration to prevent rapid increases in intrathoracic pressure which could limit venous return.

- *LLSA 2013: Manthous CA. Avoiding circulatory complications during endotracheal intubation and initiation of positive pressure ventilation. J Emerg Med. 2010; 5:622-631. full text*

#23

You are seeing a patient who has anaphylactic shock secondary to a nut allergy. Her only medication is metoprolol. You have already administered antihistamines, corticosteroids, epinephrine, large volumes of crystalloid, but despite this, the patient remains hypotensive and continues to wheeze, while developing bradycardia. What other adjunctive therapy would be the best choice to administer?

A. Prayer

B. Glucagon

C. Atropine

D. Isoproterenol

#23

Answer: B

Although prayer may be useful, no randomized trials have assessed its effects. Glucagon, can have positive inotropic and chronotropic cardiac effects mediated independently of alpha and beta-receptors. Administration may be helpful in patients who are receiving beta-blockers and who do not respond to epinephrine and antihistamines. Glucagon is thought to effect positive inotropism by augmenting cAMP synthesis through a non-adrenergic pathway. The initial dose is 1mg for adults and 0.5 mg for children, and side effects include nausea, vomiting, hypokalemia, and hyperglycemia. Atropine and isoproterenol, can also be used as second-line therapy.

- *Rosen's Emergency Medicine - Concepts and Clinical Practice. 8th edition. 2013. Chapter 119: Allergy, Hypersensitivity, Angioedema, and Anaphylaxis. 1551- 1555.*

- *Momeni M. Anaphylactic shock in a beta-blocked child: usefulness of isoproterenol. Paediatr Anaesth. 2007 Sep; 17(9): 897-9.*

#24

You are about to intubate a patient with respiratory failure in the ED. What are the reasons for providing pre-oxygenation before tracheal intubation?

A. To extend the duration of safe apnea.

B. To bring the patient's saturation as close to 100% as possible.

C. To denitrogenate the residual capacity of the lungs and thereby maximize oxygen storage in the lungs.

D. To maximally oxygenate the bloodstream.

E. All of the above.

#24

Answer: E

Preoxygenation extends the duration of safe apnea and is recommended for every ED intubation. Achieving 100% oxygen saturation and denitrogenating the residual capacity of the lungs is the primary goal. Although denitrogenating and oxygenating the blood adds little to the duration of safe apnea, because oxygen is poorly soluble in the blood and the bloodstream is a comparatively small oxygen reservoir compared with the lungs, it may add 5% to oxygen reserves.

- *Weingart SD, Levitan RM. Preoxygenation and prevention of desaturation during emergency airway management. Ann Emerg Med. 2012; 59: 165-175. full text*

#25

What is the best source of high FIO2 for preoxygenation?

A. 100% facemask

B. 10 liters/minute via nasal cannula

C. 6 liters/minute of nasal cannula and a nebulizer

D. 100% facemask with an oxygen reservoir (standardly available nonrebreather in the ED)

E. Bag-valve-mask held over the patient's face

#25

Answer: D

The 100% face mask with an oxygen reservoir (standardly available nonrebreather in the ED) lacks one way valves and only provides 60-70% FIO_2 when standard 15L/minute oxygen flows through the device. There are true non-rebreather masks with one-way valves that are usually unavailable in the ED. Using a greater O_2 flow than 15L/minute with the standard ED non-rebreathers can achieve a similar 90% inhaled FIO_2 and are the preferred means of preoxygenation. Bag Valve Masks lacking one way inhalation and exhalation ports are inadequate when preoxygenating unless there is a tight seal and active ventilatory assistance.

- *Weingart SD, Levitan RM. Preoxygenation and prevention of desaturation during emergency airway management. Ann Emerg Med. 2012 Mar; 59(3): 165-75. full text*

#26

For what period of time should the patient receive pre-oxygenation?

A. 3 minutes' worth of tidal volume breathing with a high FIO2 source

B. 8 vital capacity breaths with maximal inhalation and exhalation

C. Either of the above

#26

Answer: C

Ideally, patients should receive preoxygenation until they denitrogenate the functional residual capacity (FRC) of their lungs to achieve greater than 90% end-tidal oxygen level, which is rarely measured in the ED. Thus, 3 minutes worth of tidal volume breathing is an acceptable alternative. Patients can also take 8 vital capacity breaths if they are not well enough to cooperate.

- *Weingart SD, Levitan RM. Preoxygenation and prevention of desaturation during emergency airway management. Ann Emerg Med. 2012 Mar; 59(3): 165-75. full text*

#27

Can increasing mean airway pressure augment preoxygenation?

A. Yes

B. No

C. There is no evidence to support using noninvasive positive pressure ventilation.

#27

Answer: A

CPAP masks, noninvasive positive-pressure ventilation, or PEEP valves on a bag-valve mask device should be considered for preoxygenation and ventilation during intubation at the stage of muscle relaxation. This is important in patients who cannot achieve saturations greater than 93 to 95% with high FiO_2.

- *Weingart SD, Levitan RM. Preoxygenation and prevention of desaturation during emergency airway management. Ann Emerg Med. 2012 Mar; 59(3): 165-75. full text*

#28

In what position should the patient receive preoxygenation?

A. Supine positioning

B. Sitting upright

C. 20 to 25 degree head-up position

#28

Answer: C

Patients should receive preoxygenation in a head-elevated position, and reverse trendelenburg may be used for patients who are immobilized (c-spine precautions). An additional benefit of head elevation is better laryngeal views during intubation.

- *Weingart SD, Levitan RM. Preoxygenation and prevention of desaturation during emergency airway management. Ann Emerg Med. 2012 Mar; 59(3): 165-75. full text*

#29

How long will it take for the critically ill patient to desaturate after preoxygenation?

A. 2 minutes if the patient was otherwise healthy and was breathing room air.

B. 10 minutes if the patient was otherwise healthy and was breathing a high FiO2 level.

C. 5 minutes in an obese adult breathing a high FiO2.

D. It is impossible to predict.

#29

Answer: D

Although traditional teaching has stated that if the patient is otherwise healthy and was breathing room air, they have 1 minute of safe apnea time, 8 minutes if they were breathing a high FiO_2 percentage, and 2.7 minutes if they are obese. However in the ED due to the possible effects of shunting, increased metabolic demand, anemia, volume depletion, and decreased cardiac output, the critically ill may experience much shorter times to desaturation. One paper has estimated that time to desaturation down to 85% may be as short as 23 seconds in a critically ill adult vs. 502 seconds in a healthy adult. It is therefore impossible to predict the time to desaturation, making adequate preoxygenation imperative.

- *Weingart SD, Levitan RM. Preoxygenation and prevention of desaturation during emergency airway management. Ann Emerg Med. 2012 Mar; 59(3): 165-75. full text*

- *Benumof JL, Dagg R, Benumof R. Critical hemoglobin desaturation will occur before return to an unparalyzed state following 1 mg/kg intravenous succinylcholine. Anesthesiology. 1997; 87(4): 979-982*

#30

True or False: A nasal cannula set at 15 L/minute is the most readily available means of providing apneic oxygenation during ED tracheal intubation.

A. True

B. False

#30

Answer: A

True. In passive oxygenation, alveoli take oxygen even without diaphragmatic movements or lung expansion. In the ED, the easiest and readily available device is the nasal cannula. The decreased oxygen demands of the apneic state will allow this device to fill the pharynx and allow a steady state of oxygenation to the alveoli while the patient is sedated and paralyzed. The nasal canal can also be applied under a 100% non-rebreather mask for increased preoxygenation.

. *Weingart SD, Levitan RM. Preoxygenation and prevention of desaturation during emergency airway management. Ann Emerg Med. 2012 Mar; 59(3): 165-75. full text*

#31

What is the benefit of providing manual ventilation during the apneic period?

(Choose two answers.)

A. Prevention of hypercarbia and acidemia

B. Lengthening the duration of safe apnea

C. Prevention of barotrauma

D. Increasing venous return and improving blood pressure

#31

Answer: A and B

The risk/benefit of active ventilation during the onset phase of muscle relaxation must be carefully assessed in each patient. In patients at low risk for desaturation (> 95% O_2 sat), manual ventilation is not necessary. Those at higher risk of desaturation (91-95% O2 sat) may benefit from positive pressure ventilation. In hypoxemic patients, low-pressure, low volume, low rate ventilation will be required. Regarding choice A, it is unclear if this degree of $PaCO_2$ increase will have a clinical effect except in severe metabolic acidosis and salicylate toxicity. These patients require ventilation to match their pre-intubation respiratory rate to decrease CO_2 and prevent cardiovascular collapse. Also in patients with elevated intracranial pressure, hyperventilation (as a temporizing measure) can prevent the cerebral vasodilation caused by increasing CO_2.

- *Weingart SD, Levitan RM. Preoxygenation and prevention of desaturation during emergency airway management. Ann Emerg Med. 2012 Mar; 59(3): 165-75. full text*

#32

Which paralytic agent may be preferred in patients at high risk of desaturation during airway management?

A. Succinylcholine

B. Rocuronium

C. Vecuronium

D. Pancuronium

#32

Answer: B

Paralytic choice may also play a role in the time to desaturation. The fasciculation caused by succinylcholine (a depolarizing neuromuscular blocker) may increase oxygen use. An operating room study comparing succinylcholine to rocuronium demonstrated that the time to desaturation to 95% was 242 seconds in patients receiving succinylcholine versus 378 seconds in the rocuronium group. Thus, in patients at high risk of desaturation, rocuronium may provide a longer duration of safe apnea than succinylcholine.

- *Weingart SD, Levitan RM. Preoxygenation and prevention of desaturation during emergency airway management. Ann Emerg Med. 2012 Mar; 59(3): 165-75. full text*

#33

When etomidate was used in the Sprung CL, et al. study of hydrocortisone therapy for patients with septic shock, it was found that:

A. A single dose of etomidate inhibited the metabolism of corticosteroids for 24 hours in patients who were critically ill.

B. An association between etomidate and the likelihood of adrenal suppression was found.

C. Both of the above

D. Neither of the above

#33

Answer: C

The use of etomidate for induction of anesthesia in this study (26% of patients) was similar to that in the Annane study (24%). Etomidate has a low profile of cardiovascular complications, but a single dose can inhibit the metabolism of corticosteroids for at least 24 hours in patients who are critically ill. An association between etomidate and the likelihood of adrenal hyporesponsiveness was also found in this study.

- *Sprung CL, et al. Hydrocortisone therapy for patients with septic shock. N Engl J Med. 2008; 358: 111-124. full text*

- *Annane D, et al. Effect of treatment with low doses of hydrocortisone and fludrocortisone on mortality in patients with septic shock. Journal of the American Medical Association. 2002. 288(7): 862-871. full text*

#34

The '2" in the 3-3-2 Rule refers to:

A. The distance between the patient's incisor teeth

B. The distance between the thyroid notch and the floor of the mouth

C. The distance between the thyroid notch and the chin

D. The distance between the hyoid bone and the chin

E. The distance between the floor of the mouth and the nose

#34

Answer: B

The mnemonic LEMON (Look externally, evaluate 3-3-2 rule, Mallampati, Obstruction, Neck Mobility) is helpful in judging the potential for intubation difficulty. External characteristics that may predict difficulty with intubation include significant maxillofacial trauma, limited mouth opening, and anatomical variation such as a receding chin, overbite, or as a short neck. The 3-3-2 rule evaluated the alignment of the pharyngeal, laryngeal, and oral axes.

- The distance between the patient's incisor teeth should be at least three finger breadths.
- The distance between the hyoid bone and the chin should be at least 3 finger breadths
- The distance between the thyroid notch and the floor of the mouth should be at least 2 finger breadths.

- *Rosen's Emergency Medicine - Concepts and Clinical Practice. 8th edition. 2013. Chapter 1: Airway. 1-5*
- *WikEM - Difficult Airway Algorithm http://wikem.org/wiki/Difficult_Airway_Algorithm*

#35

When evaluating patients for hypovolemia, which of the following is the most helpful sign?

A. Postural tachycardia and the inability to stand from postural dizziness

B. Supine hypotension

C. Supine tachycardia

D. Delayed capillary refill

E. Poor skin turgor

#35

Answer: A

When clinically evaluating patients for hypovolemia, postural tachycardia and the inability to stand from postural dizziness add to diagnostic decision making while supine hypotension, supine tachycardia, capillary refill, and skin turgor have no proven diagnostic role. Vital signs and orthostatic vitals are insensitive measurements for detecting hypovolemia.

Unless a patient has significant volume loss exceeding 1,000 mL of blood, supine hypotension is also insensitive. Physical examination markers traditionally thought to be associated with dehydration (eg, dry membranes, sunken eyes) appear to be helpful when multiple positive findings are present, but their absence cannot rule out dehydration.

Sinert et al. conclude that there should be a low threshold for ordering confirmatory laboratory tests (BUN, creatinine, and metabolic panel) in the evaluation of the hypovolemic patient. Inferior vena cava ultrasound was not addressed in this review but may also aid in diagnostic evaluation.

- *LLSA 2007: Sinert R, et al. Clinical assessment of hypovolemia. Ann of Emerg Med. 2005; 45: 327-329. full text*

DERMATOLOGY

#1

Differences between Staph Scalded Skin Syndrome (SSSS) and Toxic Epidermal Necrolysis (TEN) include all of the following EXCEPT:

A. SSSS almost always occurs in children and is secondary to staph infection, whereas TEN almost always occurs in adults and is precipitated by medications.

B. Mucous membrane involvement is rare in SSSS and is limited to the lips, whereas in TEN, erosive oral lesions are common.

C. Nikolsky's sign (gentle lateral stroking of the skin causes the epidermis to separate) is positive in SSSS but it is negative in TEN.

D. Although SSSS sloughs only superficial layers of the epidermis, TEN desquamates the entire thickness of the epidermis.

E. The mortality rate in SSSS is lower than that of TEN.

#1

Answer: C

In SSSS, the skin is red, warm, and very tender. Flaccid bullae that are ill-defined and hard to see desquamate in large sheets causing the classic skin peeling appearance. Gentle lateral stroking of the skin causes the epidermis to separate.

TEN is also a disease in which the skin sloughs in large sheets. Initially, the skin is diffusely painful, hot, and red. Within 24 hours, blisters and large areas of denuded skin develop; erosive sloughing lesions of the oral mucosa are common, and the Nikolsky sign is also positive. All of the other above mentioned differences are true.

- *Rosen's Emergency Medicine - Concepts and Clinical Practice. 8th edition. 2013. Chapter 129: Bacteria. 1715-1716.*
- *Rosen's Emergency Medicine - Concepts and Clinical Practice. 8th edition. 2013. Chapter 120: Dermatologic Presentations. 1567-1568.*

#2

Which of the following dermatologic terms and definitions are INCORRECTLY paired?b*(Choose two answers.)*

A. Macule — Palpable, circumscribed lesion that is flat and greater than 1 cm in diameter

B. Papule — Palpable lesion that is solid, elevated, and less than 1 cm in diameter

C. Maculopapular — Confluent, erythematous rash made up of both macular and papular lesions

D. Purpura — Papular or macular, non-blanching lesions that are due to extravasation of red blood cells

E. Nodule — Deep-seated, roundish lesion less than 1.5 cm in diameter that can involve the epidermal, dermal, and/or subcutaneous tissue

F. Plaque — A palpable elevated lesion greater than 1 cm in diameter

G. Vesicle — A distinct, elevated skin lesion that contains fluid and is less than 1 cm in diameter

H. Bullae — A vesicle that is more than 1 cm in diameter

I. Pustule — Another term for a vesicle (synonymous with it)

J. Ulcer — Loss of the epidermis and upper layer of the dermis, resulting in a depressed skin lesion

#2

Answers: A and I

A macule is a *nonpalpable* circumscribed lesion that is flat and less than 1 cm in diameter. A pustule is a vesicle that is filled with pus. All of the other terms are correctly paired with their definitions.

- Rosen's Emergency Medicine - Concepts and Clinical Practice. 8th edition. 2013. Chapter 120: Dermatologic Presentations. 1559.

#3

Strict criteria for the diagnosis of toxic shock syndrome (TSS) include all of the following EXCEPT:

A. Fever

B. Hypotension or orthostasis

C. Erythematous macular rash

D. Involvement of at least three organ systems

E. Presence of a indwelling tampon or packing material

#3

Answer: E

Strict criteria for TSS are fever, hypotension or orthostasis, an erythematous macular rash, involvement of at least three organ systems, and the presence of a Staphylococcus aureus infection. Most patients also have facial and extremity edema.

\Staph aureus produces an exotoxin (TSST-1) that is thought to be the cause of the clinical signs and symptoms. The differential diagnosis of TSS includes Rocky Mountain Spotted Fever (RMSF), scarlet fever, sepsis, Kawasaki disease, leptospirosis, Colorado tick fever, and other viral infections.

Group A streptococcus (GAS) infection has also been reported to cause TSS due to production of streptococcal pyrogenic exotoxins. The hallmark of Streptococcal TSS, first described in the mid 1980s, is relatively early onset of shock and multi-organ failure.

The currently proposed criteria for streptococcal TSS are the presence of:

1. Isolation of group A streptococci
2. Hypotension
3. At least two of the following:
    a. Renal impairment
    b. Coagulopathy
    c. Liver function test abnormalities
    d. Adult respiratory distress syndrome
    e. Soft tissue necrosis
    f. Rash (which may be generalized macular or possibly scarlatiniform and may des-

quamate).

- *Rosen's Emergency Medicine - Concepts and Clinical Practice. 8th edition. 2013. Chapter 129: Bacteria. 1714-1717.*

#4

Regarding vesiculobullous diseases, which of the following statements is FALSE?

A. Bullous erythema multiforme (EM), Stevens-Johnson syndrome (SJS), and Toxic Epidermal Necrolysis (TEN) are on a spectrum of acute, self-limited immunologic reactions causing vesicles.

B. EM is often related to Herpes Simplex.

C. The classic lesion of EM is the target lesion, a central gray wheal or bulla surrounded by concentric rings of erythema and normal skin.

D. SJS rash may be accompanied by fever, malaise, and pruritus while EM is not

E. Although the prognosis of SJS is good, the disorder may progress to an illness clinically indistinguishable from TEN with large confluent bullae and sloughing of epidermis in sheets.

#4

Answer: D

Both SJS and EM can be accompanied by fever, malaise, and other constitutional symptoms. What distinguishes SJS from EM is the involvement of at least two mucosal membranes. With SJS, erosive lesions begin on oral mucosa, lips, and bulbar conjunctiva and can extend to the pharynx, larynx, esophagus, and genital mucosa. Ocular lesions can result in corneal ulceration, panophthalmitis, and even blindness.

- *Rosen's Emergency Medicine - Concepts and Clinical Practice. 8th edition. 2013. Chapter 129: Bacteria. 1715-1716.*

- *Rosen's Emergency Medicine - Concepts and Clinical Practice. 8th edition. 2013. Chapter 120: Dermatologic Presentations. 1567-1568, 1573.*

#5

A 77-year-old man reports a five-day history of burning and aching pain in his right side and a two-day history of erythema and clusters of clear vesicles, accompanied by headache and malaise. Which of the following statements about Herpes Zoster is INCORRECT?

A. Herpes zoster can occur in anyone who has had varicella, but is more common with increasing age and in immunocompromised patients.

B. Acyclovir, valacyclovir, and famciclovir are approved for the treatment of herpes zoster. These drugs are well tolerated and have similar efficacy.

C. Older patients, especially those over 60 years of age who have severe pain at presentation, are at increased risk for more severe disease and complications.

D. Antiviral therapy is mandatory for patients presenting with herpes zoster ophthalmicus, primarily to prevent potentially sight-threatening ocular complications.

E. Adjunctive steroid therapy has been proven effective for postherpetic neuralgia.

#5

Answer: E

To reduce the duration and severity of acute symptoms, adjunctive therapy with corticosteroids can be considered in older patients who have no contraindications. The potential for severe pain with herpes zoster should not be underestimated, and aggressive pain control is necessary. No single treatment has proved effective for postherpetic neuralgia. However, the earlier antiviral therapy is initiated (ideally within 72hrs), the higher the likelihood of clinical response. Acyclovir, famciclovir, and valacyclovir have equal efficacies, although dosing is easier with valacyclovir while its expense may be greater. Antiviral therapy should always be given for patients with herpes zoster ophthalmicus to decrease the risk of ocular complications. No study has demonstrated an effect of corticosteroids on duration of postherpetic neuralgia.

- *LLSA 2006: Gnann JW, Whitley RJ. Herpes Zoster. N Engl J Med. 2002 Aug 1;347(5):340-6. full text*

#6

An otherwise healthy 40-year-old man felt feverish and noted pain and redness over the dorsum of his foot. Tender edema and erythema extended up the pretibial area consistent with cellulitis. Fissures were present between the toes. Which of the following statements about the management of cellulitis is FALSE?

A. Comorbidities, complicating factors or degree of infection should also be considered in treatment decisions.

B. Streptococci (groups A, G, and B) and S. aureus are the most frequently isolated bacterial species.

C. Bacteremia occurs in the large majority of patients and thus, blood cultures should be sent.

D. In patients with recurrent cellulitis of the leg, any fissures in the interdigital spaces caused by epidermophytosis should be treated with topical antifungal agents to prevent recurrences.

#6

Answer: C

Bacteremia is uncommon in cellulitis. Only 2-4% of blood cultures show growth, and most are positive for either Group A Streptococci or S. aureus. Other notable organisms are H. influenzae or P. multocida. Blood cultures may be indicated in patients who have cellulitis superimposed with sepsis. All of the other statements are true.

- *LLSA 2006: Swartz MN. Cellulitis. N Engl J Med. 2004 Feb 26; 350(9): 904-12. full text*

#7

The drug of choice for scabies is Permethrin (5%) cream. However, the patient states that she is allergic. Which of the following would be a contraindication to using Lindane 1%?

A. Patients with crusted scabies or extensive dermatitis

B. Persons with seizure disorder

C. Women who are pregnant

D. Women who are breastfeeding

E. All of the above

#7

Answer: E

CNS toxicity including seizure has been reported with Lindane. It should be avoided in all the above mentioned patients, as well as in infants. For extensive dermal involvement, repeated application of lindane can cause contact dermatitis.

Contraindications include:

- Premature neonates (<28 do)
- Uncontrolled seizure disorder
- Dermatitis
- Norwegian (crusted) scabies
- Initial treatment failure

- *Rosen's Emergency Medicine - Concepts and Clinical Practice. 8th edition. 2013. Chapter 120: Dermatologic Presentations. 1567-1568.*

#8

Despite the strong association between fever, rash and an infectious disease, there are a variety of noninfectious processes that cause a fever and a rash. Which of the following noninfectious processes will NOT have an associated fever?

A. Deep vein thrombosis

B. Erythema nodosum

C. Cutaneous lupus erythematosus

D. Drug reactions

E. Allergic reactions

#8

Answer: E

Allergic reactions are not associated with a fever. All of the other skin manifestations can be associated with a fever.

- *Rosen's Emergency Medicine - Concepts and Clinical Practice. 8th edition. 2013. Chapter 119: Allergy, Hypersensitivity, Angioedema, and Anaphylaxis. 1549-1551.*

#9

You are seeing a patient with extensive toxicodendron (poison ivy) dermatitis that involves the face and the genitals. Which of the following would be the best symptomatic treatment modality for this patient?

A. Topical antihistamines

B. Topical steroids

C. Barrier cream

D. Oral steroids for 14-21 days

E. Oral steroids for 5 days

#9

Answer: D

Systemic glucocorticoids, such as a course of prednisone tapered over 14 or 21 days successfully reduces the symptoms of patients with extensive poison ivy dermatitis of the face or genitals. Short courses of systemic glucocorticoids such as the six-day methylprenisolone dose pack can cause rebound dermatitis and should be avoided. Other topical treatments for dermatitis include oatmeal baths and cool compresses. Once vesicles have developed, the high potency topical steroids do little to alter the natural course of poison ivy dermatitis except for decreasing the pruritus. Oral antihistamines may provide some relief of itching and also can be used for their sedative effects.

- *Rosen's Emergency Medicine - Concepts and Clinical Practice. 8th edition. 2013. Chapter 120: Dermatologic Presentations. 1572-1573.*

#10

A patient presents to you from the hospital kitchen 10 minutes after he accidentally spilled boiling water over his left forearm. It appears that there are areas of both first degree and second degree burns that are not circumferential. You should:

A. Place ice water on the wound

B. Place ice on the wound

C. Place warm saline on the wound

D. Apply warm compresses to the wound

E. Cool the wound with cold (15 to 25 °C) tap water

#10

Answer: E

Cold water (15 to 25 °C) applied to a burn within 30 minutes of injury will reduce the pain, depth and associated scarring. Ice water, however, may increase tissue injury and should be avoided. Ice should not be applied directly to the wound.

- *Singer AJ, et al. Current management of acute cutaneous wounds. N Engl J Med. 2008 Sep 4;359(10):1037-46. full text*

#11

You are assessing a 35 year-old patient with a severe rash that you believe is either Stevens Johnson's syndrome (SJS) or toxic epidermal necrolysis (TEN). Which of the following is FALSE regarding these two entities?

A. SJS is the less severe condition, in which skin sloughing is limited to less than 10% of the body surface area.

B. Toxic epidermal necrolysis (TEN), or Lyell's syndrome, involves sloughing of greater than 30% of the body surface area.

C. Infections are the leading cause of both SJS and TEN in both adults and children.

D. Pulmonary complications of TEN may include dyspnea, hypoxia, bronchial hypersecretion, tracheobronchitis, pulmonary edema, bacterial pneumonitis, and bronchiolitis obliterans.

E. The time course of SJS/TEN, from prodrome to hospital discharge in the absence of significant complications, is typically two to four weeks.

#11

Answer: C

SJS and TEN are most often caused by medications. Approximately 50% of SJS reactions and 80% of TEN cases have a possible medication related cause. Vaccines, systemic diseases, chemical exposure and foods have been associated with both diseases as well. In children, infection plays a more common role, albeit rare. Mycoplasma and herpes virus are infectious etiologies associated with pediatric SJS and TEN.

- *Rosen's Emergency Medicine - Concepts and Clinical Practice. 8th edition. 2013. Chapter 120: Dermatologic Presentations. 1567-1568 and 1573.*

#12

You are seeing a 52 year-old patient with herpes zoster of the T8 dermatome, and he complains of pain in that region for the last day and a half. Appropriate treatment modalities include which of the following?

(Choose two answers.)

A. Acyclovir

B. Acyclovir and prednisone

C. Valacyclovir

D. Famciclovir and prednisone

E. No treatment, since he presents > 24 hours after onset of the rash.

#12

Answer: A and C

The efficacy of antiviral therapy for the treatment of herpes zoster infection has been demonstrated by multiple randomized controlled clinical trials. The three related drugs available for treatment, which all inhibit viral replication, are acyclovir, famciclovir, and valacyclovir. The goal of treatment is to decrease the incidence of postherpetic neuralgia (PHN), time to healing, pain severity, and viral shedding.

The treatment is effective if given within 72 hours of the onset of the rash. Regarding the use of steroids, there were small benefits in a few trials with the combination use of acyclovir and steroids with adverse events related to steroid use (increased skin and soft tissue infection). A meta-analysis of five placebo-controlled trials evaluating acyclovir alone compared to antiviral therapy plus steroids did not demonstrate any benefit of combination therapy on quality of life or the incidence of postherpetic neuralgia. Routine use of corticosteroids in addition to antiviral therapy is no longer recommended.

- Rosen's Emergency Medicine - Concepts and Clinical Practice. 8th edition. 2013. Chapter 130: Viral Illnesses. 1728-1729.

#13

True statements about scarlet fever include all of the following, EXCEPT:

A. The cutaneous eruption of scarlet fever is caused by a streptococcal infection at another anatomic site, usually the tonsillopharynx.

B. During the first days of infection, the edematous papillae of the tongue appear shiny and red (strawberry red tongue).

C. The onset of the rash usually occurs 2-3 weeks after the acute streptococcal infection.

D. The rash first appears on the upper trunk and axillae and then becomes generalized. It may also appear more intense at dependent sites and sites of pressure, such as the buttocks.

E. Capillary fragility is increased manifesting as hyperpigmentation in the axillary, antecubital, and inguinal areas, known as Pastia's Lines.

#13

Answer: C

The characteristic exanthem of scarlet fever is an erythematous punctate eruption occurring 1-4 days following the onset of illness. It will first be noticed on the upper trunk and axillae and then becomes generalized, although it is usually more prominent in flexural areas, such as the axillae, popliteal fossae, and inguinal folds. It may also appear more intense at dependent sites and sites of pressure, such as the buttocks. In skin creases such as the inguinal area, Pastia's Lines may be observed. There is also associated facial flushing. The rash is compared to sandpaper due to the rough texture of the skin and usually lasts for 5 days. Occasionally, there is mild desquamation, but there is no oropharyngeal or mucosal involvement.

- *Rosen's Emergency Medicine - Concepts and Clinical Practice. 8th edition. 2013. Chapter 120: Dermatologic Presentations. 1571-1572.*

#14

You are seeing a patient who has been stung by a bee. The risk of developing anaphylaxis depends most upon which of the following?

A. The size of the bee

B. The size of the bee's stinger

C. The nature of the most severe previous reaction experienced by the patient

D. The amount of cutaneous erythema

E. Whether the patient is on oral steroid treatment

#14

Answer: C

The risk of anaphylaxis with any event is dependent on the nature of the most severe previous reaction experienced by a patient. Local reactions can be treated symptomatically with nonsteroidal anti-inflammatory agents, antihistamines, and cold compresses while the definitive therapy is epinephrine.

Epinephrine should be administered as an IM injection (0.01 mg/kg; maximum, 0.3 - 0.5 mg per dose) to anyone with more than a cutaneous reaction. Although antihistamines are often added to treat cutaneous signs and symptoms, they do not reverse the underlying problem of mast cell degranulation.Other supportive measures such as supplemental oxygen, beta-agonists for bronchospasm, and intravenous fluids for hypotension are sometimes indicated. Occasionally, for a reaction that does not respond to the initial dose of epinephrine, steroids (oral or intravenous) can be added.All patients should be prescribed an epinephrine auto-injector and be taught how to use the device prior to discharge. Patients with prior reactions are more likely to have a severe or worse reaction with subsequent allergen exposures.

- *Freeman TM. Hypersensitivity to Hymenoptera stings. N Engl J Med. 2004 Nov 4;351(19): 1978-84. full text*

#15

Which of the following factors affect topical corticosteroid potency?

A. Location of topical application on the body

B. If the area is covered with an occlusive dressing

C. Whether it is an ointment, cream, or lotion

D. Whether it is an infant's skin or an adult's skin

E. Whether the skin is inflamed and has desquamation

F. All of the above

#15

Answer: F

The potency of topical corticosteroids is affected by various factors. Topical steroids cause cutaneous vasoconstriction in relation to their potency. For example, Clobetasol propionate ointment, a Class I agent is 1000 times more potent than 1% Hydrocortisone. Steroids are readily absorbed through areas of inflammation and desquamation and better penetrate the thin stratum corneum of infants than in adults. There are also anatomic differences in absorption (percentage of dose absorbed).

- Sole of foot — 0.14%
- Palm — 0.83%
- Forearm — 1.0%
- Scalp — 3.5%

Occlusive dressings will increase absorption by maintaining skin moisture, and ointment formulations promote greater absorption than creams and lotions.

- *Rosen's Emergency Medicine - Concepts and Clinical Practice. 8th edition. 2013. Chapter 120: Dermatologic Presentations. 1558-1560.*

#16

You are seeing a patient who stated that she had an allergy to penicillin. However, she was given penicillin intramuscularly for Strep pharyngitis. Fortunately, she only develops a mild urticarial rash that resolved with benadryl. What should be disclosed to the patient?

(Choose three answers.)

A. Nothing – there was no adverse outcome

B. The patient should be provided the facts about the event – the presence of error or system failure, if known.

C. The practitioner should express regret for the unanticipated outcome.

D. The practitioner should give a formal apology if the unanticipated outcome was caused by error or system failure.

#16

Answer: B, C, and D

All adverse events should be disclosed to patients at first knowledge of the occurrence. There is no increased medical-legal liability with disclosure. By engaging in patient dialogue, the doctor-patient relationship is strengthened and there is also greater coordination of care.

- *Gallagher TH, Studdert D, Levinson W. Disclosing harmful medical errors to patients. 2007 Jun 28; 356(26): 2713-9. full text*

#17

You are seeing an African American female who has recurrent abscesses and nodules in the axillary and perineal regions concerning for Hidradenitis. TRUE statements about this disease process include which of the following?

(Choose three answers.)

A. It may be more common in females and blacks.

B. Inflammation begins deep within the acinus of the sweat glands as a result of obstruction to apocrine secretions.

C. Antibiotics are the definitive therapy.

D. It has been associated with social, personal, and professional difficulties because of chronic recurrences.

#17

Answer: A, B, and D

Hidradenitis suppurativa is a disease of chronic suppurative abscesses in the apocrine sweat glands. Although clindamycin alone or in combination with rifampin may provide temporary recession of the disease, inevitable recurrence makes surgery the definitive therapy. Severe cases may improve with immunosuppressive therapy.

The axillary location is more common than the inguinal and perineal region. Staph aureus, as well as common skin anaerobes are commonly isolated. Sinus tracts and fistulas should be unroofed, although extensive debridement should not be performed in the Emergency Department. Although rare, the most serious complication of hidradenitis is squamous cell carcinoma, so pathologic examination of surgical specimens is recommended.

. *Rosen's Emergency Medicine - Concepts and Clinical Practice. 8th edition. 2013. Chapter: 137: Skin and Soft Tissue Infections. 1859.*

#18

You have just treated a 40 year-old female who appears to have had a significant anaphylactic reaction to a hymenoptera sting. You gave her 0.3 mL of epinephrine in a 1:1000 dilution IM, 50 mg diphenhydramine intravenously, and 50 mg ranitidine intravenously. TRUE statements about this patient include which of the following?

A. After one hour, these patients should have resolution of symptoms (except for mild pruritus at sting site).

B. Any patient requiring epinephrine should be observed in the ED for recurrence.

C. There is a risk of recurrence up to 72 hours.

D. All of the above.

#18

Answer: D

All of these statements are true. Patients with anaphylaxis who require a single dose of epinephrine should be observed for up to 6 hours, and those who required multiple doses of epinephrine should be hospitalized. The rate of recurrence is probably proportional to the severity of the anaphylactic reaction, and the increased risk lasts up to 72 hours. Although epinephrine should resolve symptoms within an hour, mild pruritus may persist. Wheezing can be treated with a beta-agonist. Steroids probably play little role in preventing recurrence even though they are commonly given to blunt the biphasic reaction.

- *Rosen's Emergency Medicine - Concepts and Clinical Practice. 8th edition. 2013. Chapter 119: Allergy, Hypersensitivity, Angioedema, and Anaphylaxis. 1553-1555.*

- *Grunau BE, et al. Incidence of Clinically Important Biphasic Reactions in Emergency Department Patients With Allergic Reactions or Anaphylaxis. Ann Emerg Med. 2014 Jun;63(6): 736-44.e2. full text*

#19

In the management of cutaneous wounds, which of the following problems is NOT matched with its potential solution?

A. **Post-traumatic dirty wounds** – aggressive cleaning and removal of all foreign material

B. **Missed digital nerve injury with a laceration** – careful sensory examination, assessment of two-point discrimination

C. **Burn underestimation of depth of injury** – use of standardized charts or use of patient's palm size

D. **Laceration infections** – thorough irrigation, close followup, judicious use of systemic antibiotics, use of topical antibiotics, secondary or delayed primary closure for highly contaminated wounds.

E. **Laceration with missed foreign bodies** – careful exploration with optimal lighting, adequate hemostasis, advanced imaging, as needed.

#19

Answer: C

- Underestimation of depth of injury may be prevented by frequent reassessments and follow-up by burn specialists if the burn does not heal or if it becomes infected. The true depth of the burn becomes more obvious with time. Close follow up and surveillance are important in guiding treatment. When in doubt, early consultation with a burn specialist is recommended. Overestimation of the burn body surface area percentage may be prevented by using standardized charts of the patient's palm size. In general a patient's palm equates to 1% of burn surface area.
- First-degree burns are limited to the epidermis and are erythematous and painful. Second-degree burns involve all of the epidermis and part of the underlying dermis and are classified according to the dermal depth.
- Superficial second-degree (or partial-thickness) burns involve the upper layers of the dermis and are characterized by clear blisters and oozing. These wounds are painful and blanch with pressure. Partial thickness burns usually heal within 2 weeks, with minimal scarring.
- Deep second-degree (deep partial-thickness) burns involve the deeper layers of the dermis and are often difficult to distinguish from third-degree, or full-thickness. A third-degree burn involves the entire dermis.
- Deep dermal burns are characterized by hemorrhagic blisters, are white or red and do not blanch. These burns usually require at least 3 weeks for healing and often produce hypertrophic scarring and contractures, espe-

cially in children. It is very important to distinguish between superficial second-degree burns and deeper burns (deep partial-thickness and full-thickness burns).

- Full-thickness burns may be dark brown or tan and have a leathery texture that is insensate. Circumferential burns (burns that completely encircle a limb, the neck, or the torso) can compromise perfusion, and may require an escharotomy to relieve increasing pressure and allow for distal perfusion. An escharotomy is performed by making an incision down to the subcutaneous tissue.

- *Singer AJ, et al. Current management of Acute Cutaneous Wounds. N Engl J Med. 2008 Sep 4; 359(10):1037-46. full text*

#20

The most common musculoskeletal disorders associated with HIV in the HAART era are:

A. HIV associated arthritis

B. Rheumatoid arthritis

C. Osteoporosis and osteonecrosis

D. Septic arthritis

E. Diskitis

#20

Answer: C

The most common musculoskeletal disorders associated with HIV in the HAART era are osteoporosis and osteonecrosis, usually involving the hip. Osteoporosis has increased in prevalence with the initiation of HAART, but all HIV-infected patients have an increased risk, suggesting that HIV may play a role in the osteoporotic process. Specifically, there are increased risks of lumbosacral spine and hip fractures.

Before the introduction of HAART, HIV-positive individuals manifested multiple musculoskeletal and rheumatologic issues, most commonly HIV-associated arthritis, polymyositis, and diffuse infiltrative lymphocytosis syndrome.

New musculoskeletal and rheumatologic diseases have emerged as common in the HIV-infected patients receiving HAART. Staphylococcal pyomyositis is also being seen with greater frequency in HIV-infected patients on HAART therapy with CD4 counts less than 50 cells/mL.

- *Venkat A. Care of the HIV patient in the era of highly active antiretroviral treatment. Ann Emerg Med. 2008 Sep; 52(3): 274-85. full text*

#21

You are seeing a 92 year old female who sustained a mechanical trip and fall onto her left arm. On examination, there are no deformities, but she appears to have a 6 cm skin tear. The best treatment for this type of wound would be to:

A. Suture with 4-0 nonabsorbable sutures.

B. Suture with 4-0 absorbable sutures.

C. Approximate the wound edges with surgical tapes and cover the area with a non-adherent dressing.

D. Leave uncovered to air dry.

E. Staple the wound.

#21

Answer: C

Skin tears are particularly common among patients who are receiving long-term corticosteroids and among the elderly who tend to have fragile skin. Tears can be divided into category I, II, and III depending on the degree of degree of tissue loss.

- Category I: Classified as those without tissue loss
- Category II: Classified as those with partial tissue loss
- Category III: Classified as complete tissue loss.

Category I wounds, can be approximated with surgical tape and covered with a non-adherent dressing. For both category II and III, the wounds can be managed with non-adherent dressings, such as petroleum-based gauzes, hydrogels, foams, hydrocolloids, nylon-impregnated gauzes, and silicone-coated bandages.

Skin tears of all types that are treated within 8 hours after injury can also be approximated with a cyanoacrylate-based topical adhesive.

- *Singer AJ, et al. Current management of acute cutaneous wounds. N Engl J Med. 2008 Sep 4;359(10):1037-46. full text*

#22

You are seeing a patient who has a human bite sustained during a fist fight. Which of the following should be considerations for admission for human bites of the hand?

A. Active infection

B. Penetration of joint or tendon sheath

C. Bone involvement

D. Foreign body

E. All of the above

#22

Answer: E

Consider admitting a patient with a human bite who has:

1. Bone involvement
2. Foreign body
3. Unreliable patients or poor home situation
4. Immunosuppressed

Regardless of the above, all patients should have very close followup and antibiotics.

- *Rosen's Emergency Medicine - Concepts and Clinical Practice. 8th edition. 2013. Chapter: 50: Hand. 670-672.*

EMS

#1

In the aftermath of a disaster, hospitals use an incident command system, which is a standard emergency management system that provides a flexible command and control structure to organize a response. By standardizing an organizational structure, the incident command system provides a management system that is adaptable to incidents and spans multiple agencies and jurisdictions.

At the most basic level, there are five functional elements in the organizational structure. Which of the following is NOT one of these?

A. Incident command

B. Operations

C. Planning

D. Mitigation

E. Finance

#1

Answer: D

The five functional elements of the incident command system are:

1. Incident command
2. Operations
3. Planning
4. Logistics
5. Finance

The incident command section has overall management responsibility for the incident. Each division manages various responsibilities. Operations manages the tactical activities such as law, fire and medical. Planning collects information responsible for operations. Logistics handles facilities and materials that support operations. Finance handles payment for all services and performs relevant record keeping.

- *Rosen's Emergency Medicine - Concepts and Clinical Practice. 8th edition. 2013. Chapter 193: Disaster Preparedness. 2462-2463.*

- *FEMA - Introduction to Incident Command System http://training.fema.gov/is/courseoverview.aspx?code=IS-100.b*

#2

In a multi-casualty disaster scenario, prehospital personnel will often use a simple triage and rapid treatment (START) technique that depends on a quick assessment of respiration, perfusion, and mental status. Initially, all victims who are able to walk are asked to move away from the immediate incident area. Which color-coded triage would these patients be assigned?

A. Red

B. Yellow

C. Green

D. Black

E. None of the above

#2

Answer: C

Patients who can walk and follow commands would be classified as "green." This "self triaging" allows patients who do not need immediate medical attention to walk to an area away from the disaster site. The rescuer can then evaluate the patients, quickly checking respiratory rate, pulse, and ability to follow commands and divide them into the remaining three categories:

1. Red (immediate)
2. Yellow (delayed)
3. Black (deceased)

During the START triaging process, patient care should only include opening an airway and direct pressure on an area of hemorrhage.

- *Rosen's Emergency Medicine - Concepts and Clinical Practice. 8th edition. 2013. Chapter 193: Disaster Preparedness. 2461.*

#3

A victim arrives via ambulance and the driver states that he underwent decontamination in the field. What should be done before directing him/her to the treatment area?

A. Nothing, as the victim was already decontaminated.

B. Send the patient through the hospital decontamination process.

C. Assess the adequacy and type of field decontamination to determine if additional decontamination is necessary.

D. Send the victim to be evaluated with monitoring and detection equipment.

#3

Answer: C

The hospital's decontamination team is the first line of defense against secondary contamination of coworkers in the rest of the facility. The emergency physician must determine what kind of decontamination was provided on scene by first responders or formal HAZMAT team. If field decontamination is determined to be inadequate or uncertain, the patient should proceed through the hospital's decontamination protocol.

- *Rosen's Emergency Medicine - Concepts and Clinical Practice. 8th edition. 2013. Chapter 64: Chemical Injuries. 819.*

#4

Effective hospital decontamination of hazardous substances is best done with:

A. Bleach

B. Tepid Water

C. Hydrogen peroxide

D. Saline

#4

Answer: B

Plain water is the most practical solution for decontamination of skin. Bleach can abrade and harm the skin, and hydrogen peroxide and saline are not decontamination solutions.

- *Rosen's Emergency Medicine - Concepts and Clinical Practice. 8th edition. 2013. Chapter 64: Chemical Injuries. 819.*

#5

To prevent secondary contamination of the hospital, emergency personnel may have to do all of the following EXCEPT:

A. Secure all entrances to keep people out.

B. Set up a decontamination zone.

C. Separate everyday patients from those who are contaminated.

D. Provide victims with in-hospital life saving treatment prior to decontamination.

#5

Answer: D

Contaminated victims, even those with life-threatening conditions, should not be allowed into a hospital prior to decontamination. Hospital entrances must be secured while a decontamination team is assembled and the decontamination zone is set up. Initially, the safety of personnel and the security of the hospital are of the utmost concern.

- *Rosen's Emergency Medicine - Concepts and Clinical Practice. 8th edition. 2013. Chapter 64: Chemical Injuries. 818-827.*

#6

According to the Joint Commission, hospitals are required to implement the Hospital Incident Command System (HICS) (described in question #1) as part of disaster response. Which is the one HICS position that is always filled for every incident?

A. Finance chief

B. Incident commander

C. Planning chief

D. Operations chief

E. Liaison officer

#6

Answer: B

Every incident will have an incident commander, no matter how large or small the incident. HICS positions are only activated as needed, and it is a rare incident that requires all positions to be filled.

- *California Emergency Medical Services Authority (June 2014). Hospital Incident Command System (HICS). www.emsa.ca.gov*

#7

Victims exposed to a nerve agent in the field may be given an antidote (MARK I kit) before or during the decontamination process. This antidote comes in a:

A. Glass container with aerosol that is inhaled

B. Syringe with a spring-loaded needle

C. Oral pill form

D. Powder that is applied to the skin

E. Cream that is applied to the skin

#7

Answer: B

The antidote for nerve agent exposure is called a MARK I kit, and it contains two auto-injector syringes: one with atropine - 2 mg (to counter the cholinergic effects and dry secretions) and the other with pralidoxime 600mg (2-PAM). This is one of the few medical interventions that can be given prior to or during decontamination. There is a newer formulation of the MARK I kit, the Duo-Dote that is a single autoinjector with both medications combined.

- *Rosen's Emergency Medicine - Concepts and Clinical Practice. 8th edition. 2013. Chapter 194: Weapons of Mass Destruction. 2477.*

#8

Victims of a terrorist toxic release event will need to undress as part of the decontamination process. What should happen to the clothing after they have been removed from the patient?

A. It is bagged and returned to the victims after they are cleaned through the hospital laundry system

B. The clothing is private property and the patients may keep it

C. The clothing should be destroyed and discarded in a landfill

D. It is bagged and held as evidence for law enforcement officers

#8

Answer: D

Victim clothing should be removed, bagged, and labeled with a name and kept in a safe location. The clothing is evidence of a crime and can potentially be used by law enforcement for investigation. Since the clothing is contaminated, no one should open the bag without first receiving clearance or guidance from the jurisdictional health authority.

- *Centers for Disease Control and Prevention (2005). Radiological Terrorism Emergency Management Pocket Guide for Clinicians. http://www.bt.cdc.gov/radiation/pdf/clinicianpocketguide.pdf*

#9

There has been a radiological dispersal device (RDD) explosion ("Dirty bomb") in a nearby city. There is some radiological fallout, involving Iodine-131. A family member, who lives in the fallout zone calls you and asks you about the utility of potassium iodide (KI) administration for those who have been exposed. TRUE statements about KI administration after I-131 exposure include which of the following?

(Choose three answers.)

A. The major clinical concerns after significant I-131 exposure is the risk of hypothyroidism and thyroid cancer.

B. To reduce the risk of inhalation exposure to I-131, residents of communities near a release could stay indoors. Moist towels can be laid on window sills and at the bottom of doors to reduce air infiltration.

C. It is best to administer the KI after at least 12 hours after the exposure to I-131 to have the greatest effect in preventing thyroid uptake.

D. For patients older than 40 years of age, the risk for radiation-induced thyroid cancer is extremely low, while the potential side effects of prophylaxis due to preexisting thyroid disease tend to increase.

#9

Answer: A, B, and D

Administration of potassium iodide (KI), within the first 1-2 hours after exposure, can reduce thyroid I-131 uptake by more than 90%. If administered at 3 hours, there is a 50% reduction in uptake and at greater than 4 hours after exposure there is little to no benefit.

For patients older than 40 years of age, the risk for radiation-induced thyroid cancer is extremely low, while the potential side effects of prophylaxis due to preexisting thyroid disease tend to increase. Adults over 40 therefore do not need to take potassium iodide as prophylaxis for exposure to I-131. In the United States, the FDA has recommended prophylaxis with iodine when the dose equivalent to the adult thyroid is expected to exceed 250 milliSieverts (mSv). Sale or use of KI for this purpose does not require a physician's prescription.

- *U.S. Department of Health and Human Services Food and Drug Administration Center for Drug Evaluation and Research (December 2001). FDA Potassium Iodide as a Thyroid Blocking Agent in Radiation Emergencies. http://www.fda.gov/downloads/Drugs/.../Guidances/ucm080542.pdf*

- *ATSDR - CDC. Radiation Exposure from I-131. http://www.atsdr.cdc.gov/HEC/CSEM/iodine/docs/iodine131.pdf*

ENDOCRINE

#1

You are treating a patient with diabetic ketoacidosis and the medical student wants to provide you with an explanation of diagnosis, pathophysiology, and management. Which of his statements is FALSE?

A. Fluid deficits in DKA average 5 L.

B. Elevated potassium on presentation is common; thus, supplementation should not take place until the serum potassium decreases below 3.5 mEq/L.

C. A fall in blood glucose of 75 to 100 mg/dL/h is a reasonable goal and insulin infusions should be adjusted accordingly.

D. To avoid hypoglycemia, 5% dextrose should be added to the intravenous infusion when the blood glucose level reaches 250 mg/dL; and the insulin infusion should also be reduced by half at this point.

E. Complications of DKA therapy include hypoglycemia, hypokalemia, hypophosphatemia, fluid overload, and cerebral edema.

#1

Answer: B

Supplementation of potassium should begin when the serum potassium decreases below upper limit of normal which is 5 mEq/L. Patients with normal or low potassium should receive replacement as soon as possible before insulin administration. The administration of fluids and insulin and correction of acidosis causes intracellular shifts of potassium, leaving patients with low total body potassium vulnerable to cardiac dysrhythmias and respiratory arrest. An infusion rate of 10 to 30 mEq/h will correct typical deficits within 24 hours.

- *Rosen's Emergency Medicine - Concepts and Clinical Practice. 8th edition. 2013. Chapter 126: Diabetes and Glucose Disorders. 1656-1661.*

#2

You are treating a patient with hyperosmolar hyperglycemic state (HHS) and the medical student wants to provide you with an explanation of diagnosis, pathophysiology, and management. Which of his statements is FALSE?

A. HHS is defined by the following laboratory values: serum glucose greater than 600 mg/dL, a plasma osmolarity greater than 320 mOsm/L, and generally absence of ketoacidosis.

B. There is no history of diabetes in one-third of patients who develop HHS.

C. Infection is the most common precipitating event in HHS.

D. The degree of altered mental status corresponds with the degree and rate of development of hyperosmolarity.

E. In the HHS patient who is seizing, the medication of choice is phenytoin.

#2

Answer: E

If seizures develop in patients diagnosed with HHS, the commonly used anticonvulsants are usually ineffective. Phenytoin, which inhibits the release of endogenous insulin, may further exacerbate seizures in the setting of HHS and should be avoided. Benzodiazepines should be attempted first. All of the other statements are true.

- *Levine S, Sanson T. Treatment of hyperglycaemic hyperosmolar non-ketotic syndrome. Drugs. 1989 Sep;38(3): 462-72.*

#3

A patient is seen in the ED with altered mental status, and his blood sugar is 20. Which of the following is UNLIKELY to be the etiology of his hypoglycemia?

A. Inadequate glucose availability (missed meal)

B. Increased caloric utilization

C. The patient was started on beta agonists

D. Ethanol ingestion

E. Renal failure, hepatic failure, malnutrition, and sepsis

#3

Answer: C

Aside from insulin and sulfonylureas, a number of other drugs can precipitate hypoglycemia, either at therapeutic doses or in overdose. Patients taking beta-blockers are at increased risk for severe hypoglycemia both because of a decreased counter-regulatory response and adrenergic system in the setting of hypoglycemia. Salicylate overdoses, especially in children, can precipitate hypoglycemia. Ethanol ingestion and chronic alcoholism can cause hypoglycemia in patients with or without diabetes by suppressing gluconeogenesis. Alcoholics who consume alcohol rather than food will have depletion of their glycogen stores and can develop profound hypoglycemia and alcoholic ketoacidosis.

- Rosen's Emergency Medicine - Concepts and Clinical Practice. 8th edition. 2013. Chapter 126: Diabetes and Glucose Disorders. 1655-1656.

#4

What grocery item purchased in the US routinely contains a nutritional additive that has saved countless children from proclivity to fractures, skeletal deformities, limb pain, swelling, and seizures?

A. Milk – it does a body good

B. Bread – thiamine and carbohydrates are important cofactors for enzymatic reactions

C. Bottled water – fluoride and chlorine are necessary for neuronal membrane stability

D. Egg nog – cholesterol is important for myelin

#4

Answer: A

In the U.S., pasteurized milk is routinely fortified with vitamin D, to aid in the absorption of calcium and phosphorus. Rickets is a disease that is now relatively rare in the U.S. Vitamin D may be absorbed from a dietary source such as animal fat or be synthesized from cholesterol when one has adequate sunlight exposure. The final active metabolite is synthesized in the liver. Drugs that employ hepatic metabolism, such as phenobarbital and phenytoin, may affect liver metabolism of the vitamin D precursor and lead to rickets. Poor phosphate absorption (or excess secretion) drains the bones' hydroxyapatite stores and slowly leads to demineralized bones. Presenting features include skeletal deformities such as bowing of the extremities, rachitic rosary, and pathologic fractures; patients may have poor dentition and late eruption. Treatment includes replenishing electrolytes and starting vitamin D therapy, either with daily PO or a "jump start" IM dose of ergocalciferol, 50,000 to 100,000 IU IM.

- *Calvo M, Whiting S, Curtis, B. Vitamin D fortification in the United States and Canada: current status and data needs. Am J Clin Nutr. 2004; 80(suppl): 1710S–6S. full text*

#5

You are managing a patient that you suspect has thyroid storm. Which of the following is FALSE?

A. Inorganic iodine (Lugol's solution or SSKI) should be administered 1 hour before the administration of the thionamide, PTU.

B. PTU is the drug of choice in thyroid storm because (unlike methimazole) PTU reduces the peripheral conversion of T4 and it functions to decrease hormone synthesis.

C. In patients with an anaphylactic reaction to iodine solutions, lithium carbonate or ipodate (Oragrafin, an alternative radiocontrast agent) can be administered, which inhibits peripheral T4 conversion in addition to blocking thyroid hormone release.

D. Corticosteroids function to decrease peripheral conversion of T4 and inhibits release of hormone from the thyroid gland. Also, steroids can treat a relative adrenal insufficiency that often occurs concomitantly with thyroid storm.

E. Beta blockers are a cornerstone of therapy, and propranolol has been the agent of choice because it inhibits adrenergic overreactivity and blocks conversion of T4.

#5

Answer: A

Inorganic iodine (Lugol's solution) can be administered an hour after PTU administration. If administered before PTU, thyroid storm may be precipitated. When given after PTU, the large dose of iodine decreases the organification of thyroglobulin. Lithium carbonate may also be administered instead of inorganic iodine.

- *Rosen's Emergency Medicine - Concepts and Clinical Practice. 8th edition. 2013. Chapter 128: Thyroid and Adrenal Disorders. 1683.*

#6

You suspect that a patient you are treating in the ED has myxedema coma. Which of the following statements is FALSE regarding this entity?

A. Most patients will have signs and symptoms of hypothyroidism prior to developing myxedema coma.

B. The principal clinical features of myxedema coma are hypothermia and altered mental status, although a normal temperature is seen in 20% of patients.

C. The respiratory rate is usually reduced due to a diminished ventilatory drive, and CO2 narcosis can result.

D. An ECG most often demonstrates sinus tachycardia.

E. The treatment of myxedema coma is based on two principles: replacing thyroid hormone and identifying the precipitant event.

#6

Answer: D

An ECG most commonly demonstrates sinus bradycardia, although transient third degree heart block has been reported. Other ECG abnormalities include low voltage QRS complexes. The treatment of myxedema coma is based upon replacing thyroid hormone in the form of IV levothyroxine and identifying the precipitating cause. Since bacterial infection is the most common cause, it should be presumed to be present until proven otherwise and patients should have a full infectious workup, volume resuscitation, and administration of broad spectrum antibiotics.

- *Rosen's Emergency Medicine - Concepts and Clinical Practice. 8th edition. 2013. Chapter 128: Thyroid and Adrenal Disorders. 1683.*

#7

First line treatment modalities for myxedema coma may include all of the following, EXCEPT:

A. Levothyroxine 300-500 mcg IV followed by 50-100 mcg IV/PO per day

B. IV fluids, vasopressors, and mechanical ventilation as needed

C. Immediate invasive rewarming measures, including pleural and peritoneal infusion

D. Hydrocortisone 50-100 mg IV or dexamethasone 6mg IV

E. Treat underlying precipitants with special attention to a potential infectious etiology.

#7

Answer: C

Peripheral vasoconstriction and low intravascular blood volumes present in myxedema coma make rapid rewarming potentially hazardous. Rewarming should take place with blankets and elevated ambient room temperatures. Invasive warming mechanisms should not be the first line therapy. Aggressive rewarming may cause hypotension due to peripheral vasodilation in a patient with an already low intravascular volume. Rewarming the core first can prevent the after-drop phenomenon.

- *Rosen's Emergency Medicine - Concepts and Clinical Practice. 8th edition. 2013. Chapter 128: Thyroid and Adrenal Disorders. 1688.*

#8

All of the following statements regarding myxedema coma are true, EXCEPT:

A. The diagnosis carries a mortality rate of 30-60%.

B. Advanced age and core temperature less than 90ºF is a poor prognostic sign.

C. Bradycardia, hypotension, and concomitant sepsis or myocardial infarction increase mortality.

D. Hyponatremia < 135 should be treated with hypertonic saline.

E. Hypoglycemia may result from concomitant adrenal insufficiency and therapy with dexamethasone and stress dose steroids is indicated.

#8

Answer: D

Hyponatremia should be treated if the level is less than 120 mEq/L. However, hyponatremia usually resolves with levothyroxine therapy alone. Immediate hypertonic saline is indicated in the presence of active seizures.

- *Rosen's Emergency Medicine - Concepts and Clinical Practice. 8th edition. 2013. Chapter 128: Thyroid and Adrenal Disorders. 1687-1688.*

#9

A 70 kg male nursing home patient with sepsis is found to have a sodium of 165 mEq/L. All of the following are true statements about hypernatremia EXCEPT:

A. His free water deficit is calculated to be 10L.

B. Many nursing home patients who develop hypernatremia have deceased access to free water and are hypovolemic.

C. Hypovolemic hypernatremia patients should receive 0.9% normal saline (154 mEq/L) until they are euvolemic and can then be started on hypotonic fluids.

D. Hypervolemic hypernatremia patients may require diuretic therapy in addition to free-water replacement.

E. Diabetes insipidus causes euvolemic hypernatremia.

#9

Answer: A

His free water deficit is 7.5L and is calculated as follows:

TBW = (0.6) x (usual body weight)

TBW * [(Actual sodium – desired sodium)/desired sodium] = 0.6 x 70 [(165-140)/140] = 7.5L

For hypovolemic hyponatremia normal saline can be started initially and then titrated to a hypotonic solution as correction progresses. The majority of nursing home patients who develop hypernatremia have decreased mobility and decreased access to free water.

- *Rosen's Emergency Medicine - Concepts and Clinical Practice. 8th edition. 2013. Chapter 125: Electrolyte Disorders. 1641-1642.*

#10

Which of the following statements about hypernatremia are TRUE?

A. Mental status changes with hypernatremia range from irritability to lethargy, confusion, delirium, seizures, and coma.

B. Recommended serum sodium correction rate is 10-12 mEq/day

C. Central nervous system hemorrhage into the subarachnoid, intracerebral, and subdural space is seen in severe cases and is thought to be due to tearing of bridging veins as they are stretched by shrinkage of brain volume.

D. As with hyponatremia, the severity of symptoms correlates both with the severity of the hypernatremia and the rate at which it develops.

E. Patients with hypovolemic hypernatremia exhibit signs of dehydration, such as tachycardia, orthostasis, dry mucous membranes, diminished skin turgor, oliguria, and azotemia.

F. All of the above

#10

Answer: F

All of the above statements are true. It is important to slowly correct hypernatremia at a rate of 10-12 mEq/day. In hypernatremia, muscle tone tends to be increased, as are deep tendon reflexes. Note that there are renal and non-renal causes of hypovolemic hypernatremia. Non-renal causes include excessive sweating, vomiting, diarrhea, and decreased free water intake. The urine sodium is usually less than 10 mEq/L. Renal causes include post-obstructive, osmotic, therapeutic diuresis or cerebral salt wasting syndrome. The urine sodium is usually greater than 20 mEq/L.

- *Rosen's Emergency Medicine - Concepts and Clinical Practice. 8th edition. 2013. Chapter 125: Electrolyte Disorders. 1641-1642.*

#11

Diabetic Ketoacidosis (DKA) and hyperosmolar hyperglycemic state (HHS) may be distinguished by which of the following:

A. Presence of ketoacidosis

B. Degree of hyperglycemia

C. Degree of hypokalemia

D. Degree of hypophosphatemia

E. Degree of hypocalcemia

#11

Answer: A

DKA and HHS differ clinically according to the presence of ketoacidosis and the degree of hyperglycemia. In DKA, ketoacidosis is the major finding and serum glucose is generally below 800 mg/dL (44 mmol/L). In pure HHS, there should be no appreciable ketoacid accumulation. The serum glucose concentration frequently exceeds 1000 mg/dL (56 mmol/L), and the serum osmolality may reach 380 mosmol/kg. In the most severe cases, altered mental status is present. Significant overlap between DKA and HHS, however, occurs in more than one-third of patients.

- *Rosen's Emergency Medicine - Concepts and Clinical Practice. 8th edition. 2013. Chapter 126: Diabetes and Glucose Disorders. 1656-62.*

#12

The preferred method of measuring the degree of ketonemia in DKA is through measuring:

A. Serum beta-hydroxybutyrate

B. Serum acetoacetate

C. Serum acetone

D. Urine dipstick for ketones

E. Urine pH

#12

Answer: A

Direct measurement of beta-hydroxybutyrate in the blood is the most accurate means of detecting the ketonemia in DKA. Urine dipsticks detect acetoacetate and acetone but do not identify beta-hydroxybutyrate. During insulin therapy, beta-hydroxybutyrate is converted to acetoacetate and as treatment progresses, a greater number of ketones will be detected on urine dipstick even though the ketonemia is resolving. Resolution of DKA should never be based on resolution of ketonuria but rather on normalization of the serum bicarbonate concentration (to assess correction of the metabolic acidosis) and the serum anion gap (to assess correction of the ketoacidemia).

- *Rosen's Emergency Medicine - Concepts and Clinical Practice. 8th edition. 2013. Chapter 126: Diabetes and Glucose Disorders. 1658.*

#13

In managing DKA, the American Diabetic Association (ADA) suggests that intravenous insulin infusion can be tapered and a multiple dose subcutaneous insulin schedule can be started in patients who meet all of the following, EXCEPT:

A. Serum glucose below 200 mg/dL (11.1 mmol/L)

B. Serum anion gap less than the upper limit of normal for the local laboratory

C. Normalization of serum osmolarity

D. Venous pH >7.30

E. Serum bicarbonate ≥15 mEq/L

#13

Answer: C

DKA is resolved when the ketoacidosis resolves, as evidenced by normalization of the serum anion gap (less than 12 mEq/L) and the serum bicarbonate. Ketonemia and ketonuria may persist for more than 36 hours due to the slower removal of acetone. Since acetone is biochemically neutral, such patients have a ketosis without an associated acidosis.

The ADA guidelines suggest that the intravenous insulin infusion can be tapered, and a multiple-dose subcutaneous (SC) insulin schedule started, in patients who meet the following goals:

1. Serum glucose below 200 mg/dL (11.1 mmol/L)
2. Serum anion gap <12 mEq/L (or less than the upper limit of normal for the local laboratory)
3. Serum bicarbonate ≥15 mEq/L
4. Venous pH >7.30

- *Kitabchi A, et al. Hyperglycemic Crises in Adult Patients With Diabetes. Diabetes Care. 2009 Jul; 32(7):1335-43. full text*

#14

The most common complications in managing/treating diabetic ketoacidosis (DKA) and hyperglycemic hyperosmolar syndrome (HHS) are:

A. Hyperglycemia and renal failure

B. Hypoglycemia and hypokalemia

C. Hyperglycemia and hyperkalemia

D. Cerebral edema

E. Cardiogenic pulmonary edema

#14

Answer: B

The most common complications of the treatment of DKA and HHS are hypoglycemia and hypokalemia. Incidence is reduced with frequent monitoring of blood glucose, slow titration of insulin drips, avoidance of bolus insulin dosing, and careful monitoring of serum potassium. Hyperglycemia may result from interruption or discontinuation of intravenous insulin without prior coverage with subcutaneous insulin. Cerebral edema, although rare, is more likely in DKA (not HHS). It is primarily a disease of children and almost all affected patients are below the age of 20 years. Hypoxemia and rarely noncardiogenic pulmonary edema can complicate the treatment of DKA.

- *Kitabchi A, et al. Hyperglycemic Crises in Adult Patients With Diabetes. Diabetes Care. 2009 Jul; 32(7):1335-43. full text*

#15

In patients with DKA, the potassium should be repleted if:

A. Less than 7.5

B. Less than 7.0

C. Less than 6.5

D. Less than 6.0

E. Less than 5.0

#15

Answer: E

Patients with DKA or HHS typically have a marked degree of potassium depletion due to both renal and, in some patients, gastrointestinal losses. Potassium redistributes from the cells into the extracellular fluid, causing the initial serum potassium concentration elevation. However, insulin reverses this phenomenon. Intravenous potassium repletion should be initiated when the serum potassium concentration is ≤5.0 mEq/L. Patients with an initial serum potassium below 3.3 mEq/L should receive aggressive fluid and potassium replacement prior to treatment with insulin to prevent initial worsening of the hypokalemia.

- *Kitabchi A, et al. Hyperglycemic Crises in Adult Patients With Diabetes. Diabetes Care. 2009 Jul; 32(7):1335-43. full text*

#16

Findings suggestive of hypoparathyroidism include all of the following EXCEPT:

A. Oily, thickened skin due to poor vitamin D absorption

B. Carpal spasm on overinflation of blood pressure cuff and facial twitch on zygoma percussion

C. Papilledema and lenticular cataracts

D. Oral thrush and steatorrhea

#16

Answer A

The signs and symptoms of hypoparathyroidism are the same for hypocalcemia:

1. Chvostek's and Trousseau's signs.
2. Dry skin.
3. Brittle hair and nails.
4. Malabsorption.

Chronic hypoparathyroidism may present with papilledema, cataracts, and below normal intelligence. Treatment for hypoparathyroidism is the same as for hypocalcemia, including replacement of calcium and magnesium if needed. Long-term therapy includes oral calcium and vitamin D. Hypoparathyroidism is rare in children. It may be associated with DiGeorge's syndrome, thyroid surgery and local radiation, to name a few.

- *Rosen's Emergency Medicine - Concepts and Clinical Practice. 8th edition. 2013. Chapter: 125: Electrolyte Disorders. 1647.*

#17

You are seeing a patient who underwent a parathyroidectomy a few days ago and presents with symptoms consistent with hypocalcemia. Which of the following are reasonable management interventions?

A. Obtain a 12 lead ECG to rule out QTc prolongation, particularly in patients with underlying heart disease.

B. Infuse one 10 ml ampule of calcium gluconate over 2 minutes in symptomatic patients with confirmed hypocalcemia, repeating up to 3 doses and initiating a continuous infusion if the patient has persistent or recurrent symptoms.

C. Measure and replace magnesium when the serum magnesium level drops below 1.0 mEq/L.

D. Exclude pseudo-hypocalcemia by confirming the ionized calcium level or adjusting the serum calcium level for hypoproteinemia.

E. All of the above

#17

Answer: E

All of the above statements are true. The most common cause of a low serum calcium level is pseudohypocalcemia due to reduced serum protein states. The vast majority of cases of true hypocalcemia are due either to an insufficiency in the production of either PTH or vitamin D deficiencies. Hypocalcemia can also be caused by chelation of anions by hyperphosphatemia or large citrate loads from transfusions, sequestration from rhabdomyolysis during muscle cell damage, and saponification in cases of severe pancreatitis.

- *Rosen's Emergency Medicine - Concepts and Clinical Practice. 8th edition. 2013. Chapter 125: Electrolyte Disorders. 1647.*

#18

Regarding hypophosphatemia, which of the following statements is FALSE?

A. All disease states presenting with alkalosis or catecholamine excess can have some degree of hypophosphatemia.

B. Hypophosphatemia is commonly seen in alcoholics and patients with diabetic ketoacidosis.

C. Intravenous phosphate is indicated for those who have a serum phosphate concentration of <2 mg/dL.

D. Asymptomatic patients with mild-to-moderate hypophosphatemia can be treated orally as outpatients with sodium phosphate or potassium phosphate.

E. Serum phosphate may drop precipitously once patients with malnutrition or acidosis are treated.

#18

Answer: C

IV phosphate therapy should be initiated for symptomatic patients with serum phosphate levels less than 1 mg/dL – all others may have phosphate replaced orally. Phosphate is a crucial element in cellular metabolism for processes such as oxidative phosphorylation and glycolysis, and thus, symptoms are related to impaired skeletal and myocardial muscle function. Additionally, it can cause decreased 2,3 DPG in red blood cells, leading to a decrease in hemoglobin oxygen release in the myocardium and CNS, which may lead to altered mental status and encephalopathy. In patients with severe malnutrition, refeeding can cause phosphate to drop rapidly as insulin production causes causing intracellular shifts.

- *Rosen's Emergency Medicine - Concepts and Clinical Practice. 8th edition. 2013. Chapter 125: Electrolyte Disorders. 1648-1649.*

#19

Regarding hyperkalemia and succinylcholine, which of the following statements is FALSE?

A. When hyperkalemia occurs, it may occur within minutes after administration of succinylcholine and may be severe and fatal.

B. In a patient who has a greater than 10% body surface area (BSA) burn, the patient's vulnerability to succinylcholine begins immediately after the inciting injury or burn.

C. If the duration of burn, trauma, stroke, spinal cord injury is unknown and the patient is at risk for hyperkalemia, then favor a nondepolarizing neuromuscular blocking agent such as rocuronium.

D. In patients who have chronic denervation syndromes (such as ALS and MS), avoid the use of succinylcholine.

E. Succinylcholine is not contraindicated in renal failure but probably should not be used in patients known to have hyperkalemia if a non-depolarizing agent is available.

#19

Answer: B

A patient's vulnerability to succinylcholine-induced hyperkalemia does not begin until at least 5 days after the inciting injury or burn. The other statements are true. Rocuronium in 1.2 mg/kg offers similar onset and intubating conditions as succinylcholine but does have a longer duration of action.

- *Rosen's Emergency Medicine - Concepts and Clinical Practice. 8th edition. 2013. Chapter 1: Airway. 14.*
- *Reuban Strayer - Rocuronium vs. Succinylcholine. http://vimeo.com/8734733*

#20

Which of the following is not a feature of congenital hypothyroidism?

A. Unexplained diarrhea and malabsorption

B. Coarse facial features and large tongue

C. Constipation

D. Hoarse cry

#20

Answer: A

If not detected on neonatal screening, newborns may present in the first month or two of life with subtle and nonspecific signs and symptoms of congential hypothyroidism, such as hypoactivity, poor feeding, constipation, and prolonged jaundice. Prompt diagnosis and treatment are essential to preventing growth and mental retardation. Treatment is with L-thyroxine, at 10-15 mcg/kg/day. These children need close outpatient monitoring and follow-up.

- *Stoll C, et al. Congenital anomalies associated with congenital hypothyroidism. Ann Genet. 1999; 42(1):17-20.*

#21

Which of the following groups of patients would be more likely to die or have permanent brain damage after developing hyponatremia-induced osmotic demyelination?

A. Elderly male patient who is treated with beta blockers for hypertension

B. Male infant.

C. Elderly adult female

D. Premenopausal women

E. All of the above have the same predisposition to neurologic dysfunction with osmotic demyelination

#21

Answer: D

For reasons that are not well understood, premenopausal women appear to be at greater risk for severe hyponatremic symptoms and at much greater risk (up to 25-fold when compared to men) for residual neurologic injury following symptomatic hyponatremia.

In one epidemiologic study of postoperative patients, women were as likely as men to develop hyponatremia (defined as a plasma sodium concentration ≤128 mEq/L). However, women comprised 97% of cases of death or irreversible brain damage after an episode of symptomatic hyponatremia even if the plasma sodium concentration were raised at an appropriate rate. There may be a hormonally-mediated processes that predisposes premenopausal women to poor osmotic adaptation.

- *Ayus JC, Wheeler JM, Arieff AI, Postoperative hyponatremic encephalopathy in menstruant women. Ann Intern Med. 1992 Dec 1; 117(11): 891-7.*

#22

You are seeing a nursing home patient with hypernatremia (160 mg/dL). The patient has an altered mental status at baseline, and he is apparently more altered than usual (he normally responds to command but is not able to verbalize). What is the maximum rate by which you should correct his serum sodium?

A. 5 mEq/hr

B. 3 mEq/hr

C. 1 mEq/hr

D. 0.25 mEq/hr

E. 0.5 mEq/hr

#22

Answer: E

As in hyponatremia, the cerebral adaptation in hypernatremia has important clinical consequences. Chronic hypernatremia is much less likely to induce neurologic symptoms. Correction of chronic hypernatremia must occur slowly to prevent rapid fluid movement into the brain and cerebral edema. Rapid correction can lead to seizures and coma. As a result, the rate of correction in asymptomatic patients **should not exceed 12 mEq/L per day**, which represents an average of 0.5 mEq/L per hour. There are no definitive clinical trials, but data in children suggest that the maximum safe rate at which the plasma sodium concentration should be lowered is by ≤0.5 mEq/L per hour and no more than by 12 mEq/L per day.

Hypernatremia initially causes fluid to leave the brain resulting in symptoms related to the cerebral contraction. Brain volume restores within 3 days of sodium correction. Rapidly lowering the plasma sodium concentration once cerebral contraction has occurs can cause a pathologic increase in brain size.

- *Rosen's Emergency Medicine - Concepts and Clinical Practice. 8th edition. 2013. Chapter 125: Electrolyte Disorders. 1642.*

- *Kim, S. Hypernatemia: Successful Treatment. Electrolyte Blood Press. 2006 Nov; 4(2): 66–71. full text*

#23

In your 60 kg female patient with hypernatremia and a serum sodium of 168 mEq/L, what is her free water deficit?

A. 10.2 liters

B. 8 liters

C. 6 liters

D. 3.4 liters

E. 2 liters

#23

Answer: C

$$\text{Water deficit} = \text{TBW} \times \left(\frac{\text{plasma [Na+]}}{140} - 1\right)$$

The total body water is normally about 60 and 50% of lean body weight in younger men and women, respectively, and is somewhat lower in the elderly (about 50 and 45% in men and women, respectively). Thus, in a 60 kg woman with a plasma sodium concentration of 168 mEq/L, total body water is about 50% of body weight and the water deficit can be approximated from:

Water deficit = 0.5 x 60 ([168/140] - 1) = 6 liters

This formula estimates the amount of positive water balance required to return the plasma sodium concentration to 140 mEq/L. Then, when calculating the amount of free water to give (either intravenously, as dextrose in water, or orally if the patient is able to drink), insensible losses and some part of urine and gastrointestinal losses must be added to the calculation.

- *Rosen's Emergency Medicine - Concepts and Clinical Practice. 8th edition. 2013. Chapter 121: Electrolyte Disorders. 1641-42.*

#24

A 60kg female patient is seizing and has a serum sodium of 113 mEq/L with no underlying history of seizures. What should be the treatment of her hyponatremia?

A. Hypertonic saline 3% - 290 ml over 2 hours

B. Normal saline 3% - 50 ml over 30 minutes

C. Phenytoin 1 gram

D. Hypertonic saline 3% - 1000 ml IV bolus

E. Hypertonic saline 3% - 750 ml over 2 hours

#24

Answer: A

To acutely stop seizure activity in a hyponatremic patient, you will need to raise the serum sodium by 5 mEq/liter of total body water (TBW). **290 mL of hypertonic saline will allow for an increase serum sodium by 5 mEq/L** (could be administered as 145 mL/h for 2 h). Alternatively 100ml of 3% saline can be pushed IV to attempt immediate seizure cessation.

- The Sodium Requirement (mEq) = TBW x (Desired Na - Serum Na) where TBW = Body Weight x 0.6 (for men) or 0.5 (for women).
- 3% hypertonic saline has 513 mEq of Na per liter.
- Volume of Hypertonic Saline = Na Requirement (mEq)/Infusate Na Concentration (mEq/L)
- In a 60-kg woman with serum sodium level of 113 mEq/L, the amount required is 0.5x60x5=150mEq of Na. 150/513 = 292ml of 3% hypertonic saline.

In general, 200-400 mL of 3% NaCl is reasonable dose in most adult patients with severe symptomatic hyponatremia.

- *Moritz ML, Ayus JC. 100cc 3% sodium chloride bolus: a novel treatment for hyponatremic encephalopathy. Metab Brain Dis. 2010 Mar; 25(1): 91-6.*
- *EmCrit.org - Severe Hyponatremia http://emcrit.org/podcasts/hyponatremia/*

#25

A 42 year-old woman is brought to the ED for "med clearance." Her husband says that she has been "acting like a fool." The husband wants his wife admitted to the psychiatric ED. The patient is quiet, then laughs briefly and inappropriately. On further questioning, the patient states that she has had abdominal pain of unclear duration. Her review of systems is pan-positive: vague complaints of intermittent nausea, constipation, "everything hurts", and she may have had some blood in her urine "awhile back". Her vital signs are normal, and her exam is significant for hyperreflexia. Since metabolic and toxicologic causes are on your differential, you order an ECG, which shows normal sinus rhythm at 70 bpm, no pre-excitation, no block, QRS at 100 msec, and QTc at 300msec. How do you proceed?

A. Obtain a urine toxicology screen and call social work.

B. Check electrolytes and serum calcium, administer IV fluids and, admit for a further metabolic workup.

C. Do a thorough history and physical and call psychiatry.

D. Order an abdominal ultrasound, start giving oral contrast, and re-examine her to determine if she needs a CT abdomen and pelvis.

#25

Answer: B

This vague presentation illustrates the difficulty of both medical clearance and diagnosis of hyperparathyroidism. Hyperparathyroidism is most commonly diagnosed in middle age. It is uncommon in children, but there may be a family history of the same, and there is an association with multiple endocrine neoplasia (MEN) types I and II. The presentation of hyperparathyroidism is basically the presentation of hypercalcemia, without apparent cause: weakness, anorexia, vomiting, constipation, personality changes, renal colic ("Stones, Bones, Groans, and Psychic Overtones"). Associated signs and findings include hypertension, shortened QTc, and polyuria. The hyperreflexia should be a clue that there is an organic cause for her altered mental status. X-rays may show demineralization and rarely osteitis fibrosa cystica (calcified bone is replaced by fibrous tissue). Treatment includes aggressive volume repletion, and may include furosemide after IV fluids depending on the degree of her hypercalcemia.

- *Rosen's Emergency Medicine - Concepts and Clinical Practice. 8th edition. 2013. Chapter 125: Electrolyte Disorders. 1645-1646.*

#26

Which of the following is TRUE in Diabetes Insipidus (DI)?

(Choose two answers.)

A. Most cases of central DI present in the newborn period.

B. Patients may present with polyuria, polydipsia, and urinary ketones.

C. Most cases of nephrogenic DI occur in males in infancy.

D. Criteria for diagnosis include low urinary specific gravity and a high serum sodium.

#26

Answer: B and C

Diabetes Insipidus is caused by an inability to concentrate urine, and may be central (deficiency of antidiuretic hormone production (ADH) from the posterior pituitary) or nephrogenic (renal unresponsiveness to ADH secretion).

Central DI may present at any age. The vast majority of cases of nephrogenic DI in children are due to X-linked recessive inheritance. Newborns present primarily with signs and symptoms of volume depletion. Older children may have the additional history of compensation by increasing oral fluid intake and waking up in the middle of the night due to thirst.

Specific diagnostic criteria include:

1. Elevated serum osmolality > 300 mOsm/L
2. Elevated serum sodium > 145 mmol/L
3. Dilute urine osmolality < 600 mmol/L.

Treatment includes volume repletion and DDAVP. The dose of DDAVP for children 3 mo - 12y is 5-30 mcg/day (divided twice daily); the adult dose is 10-40 mcg/day (divided twice daily).

- *Makaryus AN, Mcfarlane SI. Diabetes insipidus: diagnosis and treatment of a complex disease. Cleve Clin J Med. 2006; 73(1): 65-71. full text*

#27

You are seeing patient who is brought in by paramedics and family for lethargy and confusion, The family reports that the patient underwent I-131 therapy several years ago for hyperthyroidism and is on thyroid replacement therapy. The family just returned from a 1 week ski vacation and found the patient in her bed confused and cold. All of the following may be found in this patient with myxedema coma EXCEPT:

A. Hypotension

B. Bradycardia

C. Hyponatremia

D. Hyperglycemia

E. Pericardial effusion

#27

Answer: D

Hypoglycemia, rather than hyperglycemia, may be caused by hypothyroidism alone or, more often, by concurrent adrenal insufficiency due to autoimmune adrenal disease or hypothalamic-pituitary disease. There is also decreased gluconeogenesis. Hyponatremia is present in approximately one-half of patients with myxedema coma and further complicates the differential diagnosis if the history of thyroid disease is not known. Most, but not all, patients have an impairment in free water excretion due to inappropriate excess vasopressin secretion or impaired renal function. Myxedema coma is associated with bradycardia, decreased myocardial contractility, a low cardiac output, and sometimes hypotension.

- *Rosen's Emergency Medicine - Concepts and Clinical Practice. 8th edition. 2013. Chapter: 128: Thyroid and Adrenal Disorders. 1687.*

#28

You are seeing an alcoholic patient who is brought in by the family for altered mental status, gait ataxia, and oculomotor dysfunction. Which of the following statements is FALSE about this condition?

A. The classic triad consists of gait ataxia, ophthalmoplegia, and encephalopathy.

B. The first management priority after the ABC's is to administer thiamine.

C. May be precipitated by administration of intravenous glucose solutions to individuals with thiamine deficiency.

D. Only alcoholics can develop this entity.

#28

Answer: D

Wernicke's encephalopathy (WE) and Korsakoff's amnesic syndrome (KS) are, respectively, acute and chronic brain disorders that result from thiamine deficiency. WE is most often associated with alcoholism but can also occur in other situations including malnutrition from any cause (particularly at the time of refeeding) and in dialysis patients. WE produces hemorrhagic necrosis in midline brain structures causing altered mental status, nystagmus and ataxia. The classic triad is found in less than a third of patients, and encephalopathy occurs most commonly.

While laboratory measurements and neuroimaging may provide clues to the diagnosis, if there is suspicion for the disease in the right clinical setting, thiamine should be administered. If the patient has a thiamine deficiency, glucose administration should only occur after thiamine is administered (100mg) parenterally.

- *Rosen's Emergency Medicine - Concepts and Clinical Practice. 8th edition. 2013. Chapter: 185: Alcohol Related Disease. 2386.*

#29

You are seeing a patient with hypercalcemia. Which of the following medications could be contributing to his hypercalcemia?

A. Hydrochlorothiazide

B. Theophylline

C. Lithium

D. Vitamin A

E. Calcium

F. All of the above

#29

Answer: F

Thiazide diuretics can lower urinary calcium excretion, an effect that is useful in the treatment of patients with hypercalciuria and recurrent calcium nephrolithiasis. Theophylline toxicity has been associated with mild hypercalcemia. Hypervitaminosis A (greater than 50,000 units per day) or the administration of retinoic acid cause increases in bone resorption. A high calcium intake alone is a rare cause of hypercalcemia, because the initial elevation in serum calcium concentration inhibits both the release of parathyroid hormone (PTH) and the synthesis of calcitriol. When combined with decreased urinary excretion, however, increased intake can cause hypercalcemia. This combination occurs in two situations: chronic kidney disease and the milk-alkali syndrome. Patients receiving lithium therapy develop mild hypercalcemia, most likely due to increased secretion of PTH. The hypercalcemia usually resolves with cessation of lithium. Lithium can unmask previously unrecognized mild hyperparathyroidism or directly raise PTH levels.

- *Rosen's Emergency Medicine - Concepts and Clinical Practice. 8th edition. 2013. Chapter 125: Electrolyte Disorders. 1645-1646.*

#30

You are calculating the anion gap for a patient, and you find that it is very low (<5). Causes of a low anion gap include which of the following?

A. Multiple Myeloma

B. Hypoalbuminemia

C. Hyperkalemia, Hypercalcemia, or Hypermagnesemia

D. Lithium intoxication

E. All of the above

#30

Answer: E

The most common cause of a low anion gap (less than 7 mEq/L) is laboratory error. A verifiably low AG can be induced by a fall in the unmeasured anions (primarily due to hypoalbuminemia) or by a rise in unmeasured cations. The latter can occur with hyperkalemia, hypercalcemia, hypermagnesemia, or lithium intoxication. Multiple myeloma, which causes cationic paraprotein production, and IgG gammopathy can also cause low anion gap. With hypoalbuminemia, the expected normal values for the anion gap can be recalculated. The anion gap falls by about 2.5 mEq/L for every 1 g/dL (10 g/L) reduction in the plasma albumin concentration.

In rare cases, the anion gap has a negative value. This is most often due to a laboratory artifact in severe hypernatremia (at levels above 170 mEq/L), hyperlipidemia, or bromide intoxication. Other than direct bromide ingestion, bromide intoxication can occur in patients taking pyridostigmine bromide for myasthenia gravis. Some herbal remedies also contain bromide.

- *Berend K, et al. Physiological approach to assessment of acid-base disturbances. N Engl J Med. 2014; 371(15): 1434-45.*
- *Vasuyattakul S, et al. A negative anion gap as a clue to diagnose bromide intoxication. Nephron. 1995; 69(3): 311-3.*
- *FDA - Pyridostigmine Bromide Tablets. http://bit.ly/kaji-pyrido-bromide*

#31

You are now assessing a patient with an elevated anion gap (>20). Causes of an elevated anion gap include which of the following?

A. Metabolic acidosis due to lactic acidosis, diabetic ketoacidosis, alcoholic ketoacidosis

B. Hyperphosphatemia

C. Metabolic alkalosis

D. Significant rise in albumin concentration

E. Overproduction of an anionic paraprotein

F. All of the above

#31

Answer: F

An elevated anion gap (AG) can be produced by an increase in unmeasured anions (as in several causes of metabolic acidosis) or by a reduction in unmeasured cations. The most common causes of a metabolic acidosis with an elevated anion gap are lactic acidosis, ketoacidosis, or toxic ingestions such as aspirin, methanol, ethylene glycol, and toluene.

Reduction in unmeasured cations (hypocalcemia, hypomagnesemia) is a potential contributing factor and if present should only contribute to a few mEq/L increase in AG. Mild elevation in AG can also occur in metabolic alkalosis. Metabolic alkalosis is associated with an increase in the negative charges per albumin molecule. Since albumin is one of the main components of the normal anion gap, an increase in albumin or change in the charge of albumin increases the anion gap. Anion paraprotein production and hyperphosphatemia can also contribute to an elevated anion gap.

- *Kraut JA, Madias NE. Serum anion gap: its uses and limitations in clinical medicine. Clin J Am Soc Nephrol. 2007; 2(1): 162-74. full text*

#32

You are now seeing a patient with hyperkalemia and a potassium of 7.0 mEq/L. All of the following statements below are true EXCEPT:

A. IV calcium gluconate has an onset of action < 5 minutes.

B. IV calcium gluconate has a duration of action of 4-6 hours.

C. If the patient is on digoxin, it would be a good idea to obtain a digoxin level.

D. An ECG is essential to assess for cardiac conduction disturbances related to hyperkalemia.

E. Medications, such as calcium, insulin, glucose, and sodium bicarbonate, are temporizing measures. Definitive treatment is dialysis.

#32

Answer: B

Calcium stabilizes the myocardium by restoring a normal gradient between the threshold potential and resting membrane potential, which is elevated in hyperkalemia. One ampule of calcium chloride has approximately 3 times more calcium than calcium gluconate. Onset of action is <5 min and lasts about 30-60 min, decreasing the risk of ventricular fibrillation during that time.

Calcium should be administered in any patient with hyperkalemia and a wide QRS interval, loss of P waves, or any cardiac arrhythmias. For peaked T waves, calcium will not have any measurable effect and should not be given.

Ultimately, patients require emergent dialysis since medications such as calcium, insulin, and glucose are temporizing measures. Elimination of potassium only occurs after 72+ hrs with repeat doses of resin-binding agents (kayexalate), or over 4-6 hours with with diuresis (furosemide).

- *Rosen's Emergency Medicine - Concepts and Clinical Practice. 8th edition. 2013. Chapter 125: Electrolyte Disorders. 1637-39.*

#33

In general, therapeutic treatment options for thyroid storm is similar to that for the treatment of uncomplicated hyperthyroidism. Which of the following are differences in therapeutic management options when you are treating a patient with thyroid storm?

A. The doses of the medications are higher

B. The medications are given more frequently

C. Monitoring in an intensive care unit may be required

D. If they have a fever, then acetaminophen is preferred to aspirin

E. Some may require diuresis while others may require intravenous fluid hydration.

F. All of the above

#33

Answer: F

The therapeutic options for thyroid storm are the same as those for uncomplicated hyperthyroidism, except that the drugs are given in higher doses and more frequently. In addition, intensive care monitoring is required since the mortality rate of thyroid storm is high. Many patients require a substantial amount of fluid, while others may require diuresis because of congestive heart failure. Infection needs to be identified and treated; and hyperpyrexia should be aggressively corrected. Acetaminophen is preferable to aspirin, which can increase serum free thyroxine (T4) and triiodothyronine (T3) concentrations by interfering with protein binding.

. *Rosen's Emergency Medicine - Concepts and Clinical Practice. 8th edition. 2013. Chapter: 128: Thyroid and Adrenal Disorders. 1680-1684.*

#34

In the treatment of the patient with thyroid storm, which of the following may be administered as part of the pharmacologic treatment regimen?

A. Beta-blockers

B. Thionamides

C. Iodine

D. Glucocorticoids

E. All of the above

#34

Answer: E

The therapeutic regimen typically consists of multiple medications, each of which has a different mechanism of action:

1. A beta-blocker to control the symptoms induced by increased adrenergic tone.
2. A thionamide, such as methimazole or PTU, to block new hormone synthesis.
3. An iodine solution to block the release of thyroid hormone (after blockage of new synthesis).
4. Corticosteroids to reduce T4-to-T3 conversion and treat relative adrenal insufficiency.

Note that lithium has also been given to acutely block the release of thyroid hormone. However, its renal and neurologic toxicity limit its utility.

- *Rosen's Emergency Medicine - Concepts and Clinical Practice. 8th edition. 2013. Chapter 128: Thyroid and Adrenal Disorders. 1680-84.*

#35

The possible presence of rhabdomyolysis should be suspected in:

A. A person with myalgia and pigmenturia in a patient who can provide reliable information

B. A stuporous patient with muscle tenderness

C. A comatose patient with signs of multiple trauma

D. A comatose patient with hyperkalemia, hyperphosphatemia, or hypocalcemia

E. A person who tells you that they just completed a marathon and has severe muscle pains

F. All of the above

#35

Answer: F

The possible presence of rhabdomyolysis should be suspected in any patient who has one or more of the following:

1. Muscle tenderness
2. Evidence of pressure necrosis of the skin
3. Signs of multiple trauma or a crush injury
4. Blood chemistry abnormalities suggesting the possibility of increased cell breakdown, such as hyperkalemia, hyperphosphatemia, and/or hypocalcemia

Note that renal failure, as evidenced by an elevated serum creatinine, may or may not be present. The most common causes are muscle overuse, ischemic muscle from severe infection or sympathomimetics, alcoholism, medication side effects, hypokalemia, hypophosphatemia, severe agitation, or intrinsic muscle disorders.

- *Huerta-alardín AL, Varon J, Marik PE. Bench-to-bedside review: Rhabdomyolysis - an overview for clinicians. Crit Care. 2005; 9(2): 158-69. full text*

#36

The syndrome of inappropriate secretion of ADH (SIADH) is one of the causes of euvolemic hyponatremia. If you suspect that a patient has SIADH, you would expect to find:

A. A urine osmolarity > 350 mOsm/kg

B. A high serum osmolarity

C. A high circulating blood volume

D. All of the above

#36

Answer A

The clinical picture of SIADH is an inappropriately concentrated urine, with a low serum osmolarity and a normal circulating blood volume. Causes of SIADH include CNS disorders, pulmonary disease, drugs, stress, pain and surgery. Before the diagnosis of SIADH can be confirmed, other potential causes of euvolemic hyponatremia need to be ruled out (hypoadrenalism, hypothyroidism, renal failure, psychogenic polydipsia, etc).

- *Rosen's Emergency Medicine - Concepts and Clinical Practice. 8th edition. 2013. Chapter 125: Electrolyte Disorders. 1642-1645.*

#37

Most patients seen in the ED for hypoglycemia can be discharged. Which of the following are reasonable discharge criteria?

A. If they are a type I diabetic

B. If they are a type II diabetic

C. If they are age < 75

D. None of the above

#37

Answer: D

Some discharge criteria for hypoglycemia include the following:

1. Brief episode
2. Full neurological recovery
3. Able to eat
4. No major comorbidities that require hospital admission
5. Cause of episode found and addressed
6. Treatment plan to prevent future episodes understood by the patient
7. Accidental cause (not intentional overdose)
8. Relapse unlikely because it is not due to a long-acting insulin or oral agent
9. Able to do home glucose monitoring
10. Responsible person to be with the patient, and follow-up arranged

Hospital admission is indicated for patients failing to meet these criteria. Hypoglycemic patients with type II diabetes require hospitalization more frequently owing to the need for monitoring in patients with sulfonylurea induced hypoglycemia, poor general condition, and a higher rate of concomitant disease requiring treatment.

- *Rosen's Emergency Medicine - Concepts and Clinical Practice. 8th edition. 2013. Chapter 126: Diabetes and Glucose Disorders. 1656.*

#38

In the patient with alcoholic ketoacidosis (AKA), which of the following treatments is most important?

A. Intravenous insulin

B. Parenteral thiamine

C. Intravenous dextrose

D. Correction of electrolyte abnormalities

E. Sodium bicarbonate

#38

Answer: C

Glucose must be given to correct the underlying cause of AKA, which is primarily the lack of glucose and glycogen stores. Glucose provides an energy substrate and stimulates insulin release from the pancreatic beta-islet cells. Insulin, once released, inactivates hormone-sensitive lipase. This process leads to decreased release of free fatty acids, the substrate for ketogenesis. Thus, glucose is able to stop ketone formation. Glucose should initially be given intravenously as 5% dextrose unless the patient is significantly hypoglycemic, in which case a 50% dextrose bolus is indicated. Sodium bicarbonate is unnecessary, and the acidosis usually resolves rapidly with fluid and glucose. Insulin is unnecessary unless the patient has a known history of diabetes or persistent hyperglycemia.

- *Rosen's Emergency Medicine - Concepts and Clinical Practice. 8th edition. 2013. Chapter 185: Alcohol Related Disease. 2388.*

#39

Which of the following are clinical features of hypercalcemia?

(Choose two answers.)

A. Generalized fatigue

B. Prolongation of the QT interval

C. Diarrhea

D. Edema

E. Nephrolithiasis

#39

Answer: A and E

The clinical manifestations of hypercalcemia are nonspecific and vary widely from patient to patient. Severity of the symptoms depends on both the level of serum calcium and the rapidity of the rise. Hypercalcemia decreases neuronal conduction and causes fatigue, weakness, altered mental status, lethargy, and even coma. Hypercalcemia causes shortening of the QT interval and prolongation of the PR interval. It can also cause sinus bradycardia, and it can potentiate the effects of digoxin. Because hypercalcemia causes polyuria, dehydration, and vomiting, patients do not present with edema. Gastrointestinal manifestations include constipation and ileus, as well as nausea, vomiting, pancreatitis, and peptic ulcer disease. Hypercalcemia can also lead to nephrolithiasis and nephrocalcinosis.

- *Rosen's Emergency Medicine - Concepts and Clinical Practice. 8th edition. 2013. Chapter 128: Thyroid and Adrenal Disorders. 1645.*

ENT

#1

Regarding epistaxis, which of the following statements is FALSE?

A. Most cases of epistaxis are minor and the episode frequently terminates in the triage area with the proper application of pressure (firm grasp and pinch of the entire soft, anterior portion of the nose) for 10 to 15 minutes.

B. Anterior epistaxis typically arises from Kisselbach's plexus, also known as Little's area, an anastomotic network of vessels in the anterior portion of the nasal septum.

C. Approximately 90% of epistaxis is anterior, which means the bleeding source can be visualized in the anterior portion of the nasopharynx.

D. A patient with posterior packing should be discharged and followed up in ENT clinic in 24-48 hours.

E. Anterior nasal packing prevents normal surgical drainage of the sinuses, and patients should be placed on a first generation cephalosporin to prevent toxic shock syndrome.

#1

Answer: D

All patients with posterior packing should be admitted. Posterior packs are fraught with complications, including hypoxia, hypercarbia, exacerbation of obstructive sleep apnea, aspiration, hypertension, bradycardia, arrhythmias, myocardial infarction, and death. All of the other statements are true.

- *Roberts and Hedges' Clinical Procedures in Emergency Medicine. 6th edition. 2013. Chapter 63: Otolaryngologic Procedures. 1130-1131.*

#2

A young 20 year old male presents after he was "punched in the nose" without any associated LOC, and no difficulty breathing. On physical exam, he has some swelling and ecchymoses over the nasal bridge but no crepitus and no septal hematoma. There does not appear to be a significant deformity. All of the following are appropriate in the management of nasal fractures, EXCEPT:

A. Plain AP, lateral, and oblique radiographs of the nasal bone should be obtained.

B. If there is no misalignment, the only treatment includes ice packs and analgesia.

C. With significant deformity, the patient should be referred to a consultant as an outpatient within 5 to 7 days after swelling has subsided.

D. If the patient has a septal hematoma, a no. 11 blade should be used to incise the inferior portion of the hematoma and packed with petroleum gauze, as an undrained hematoma can lead to abscess formation or necrosis of the nasal cartilage with resultant saddle nose deformity.

E. If the patient has proven CSF rhinorrhea, then emergent reduction and fixation is indicated.

#2

Answer: A

Nasal bone fractures are often diagnosed with history and physical exam alone. Nasal films are generally deemed unnecessary as they do not affect management. Although difficult to asses due to soft tissue swelling, a missed septal hematoma can cause significant necrosis due to increased pressure on the nasal septum. Generally for significant deformities of the nasal bone, outpatient evaluation for fixation is most appropriate due to the need for swelling to subside before surgical realignment. If there is evidence of CSF rhinorrhea, in addition to need for ENT consult and reduction, advanced imaging should be performed to look for other associated facial fractures.

- *Rosen's Emergency Medicine- Concepts and Clinical Practice. 8th edition. 2013. Chapter 42: Facial Trauma. 368-369.*

#3

All of the following are characteristics of naso-orbito-ethmoid (NOE) fractures, EXCEPT:

A. Typically, this injury is caused by the bridge of the nose hitting the steering wheel or dashboard with high force or by an assault with a blunt object.

B. A decrease in the distance between the medial canthi is suggestive of this fracture.

C. There may be a flattened nasal bridge, enophthalmos, and epiphora.

D. It is important to rule out associated lacrimal system injury and recognize the NOE fractures since repair is difficult if delayed.

E. Due to the thick bones and complex anatomy, radiographic assessment is best made with a facial CT scan, rather than plain radiographs.

#3

Answer: B

The interpupillary distance (IPD) is the distance between the center of the pupils of the two eyes. In patients with a NOE fracture there will be a widening of the nasal bridge, and an increase in the distance between the medial canthi of each eye. Normal distances are 35-40 mm and an increase in this measurement (telecanthus distance) suggests a NOE fracture. Generally, a CT face will provide definitive diagnosis in the ED.

- *Rosen's Emergency Medicine- Concepts and Clinical Practice. 8th edition. 2013. Chapter 42: Facial Trauma. 368-369.*

#4

Which of the following two facial fractures impact future facial development in a child?

(Choose two answers.)

A. Mandibular condyle fracture

B. Nasal septal fracture

C. Mandibular ramus fracture

D. Zygoma fractures

E. Orbital floor fractures

#4

Answer: A and B

There are two fractures that impact future facial development in children. Mandibular condyle fractures can result in growth disturbances, deformities, and ankylosis secondary to damage of the growth centers. Displaced nasal injuries also affect future development of the naso-maxillary buttress.

- *Rosen's Emergency Medicine- Concepts and Clinical Practice. 8th edition. 2013. Chapter 42: Facial Trauma. 380.*

#5

The least commonly fractured area of the mandible is:

A. Mandibular body

B. Mandibular coronoid

C. Mandibular condyle

D. Mandibular angle

E. None of the above

#5

Answer: B

Areas of the mandible that are most commonly fractured are the mandibular condyle (18%), body (36%), and the angle (31%). Coronoid fractures account for 1% of the fractures. After nasal bone fractures, the mandible is the most commonly fractured facial bone. Due to transmission of force through its ring shape, the mandible is frequently broken in multiple locations. The first sign a clinician may notice on exam besides for pain is poor alignment of teeth with closure of the jaw.

- *Rosen's Emergency Medicine- Concepts and Clinical Practice. 8th edition. 2013. Chapter 42: Facial Trauma. 369-371.*

- *Rashid A, et al. Incidence and patterns of mandibular fractures during a 5-year period in a London teaching hospital. Br J Oral Maxillofac Surg. 2013 Dec; 51(8): 794-8*

#6

A patient presents with mouth pain after a tooth extraction. Which of the following statements about "dry socket" syndrome or alveolar osteitis is FALSE?

A. Typically, patients present 3 to 5 days following the extraction with severe localized pain.

B. It is often associated with fever, malaise, leukocytosis, and the surrounding teeth and bone may be sensitive to palpation.

C. It is due to the socket losing the protective clot prematurely, exposing the socket down to the bone.

D. Some patients complain of a foul odor or taste.

E. For management, the socket should be irrigated with warmed saline, dried thoroughly, and packed with soaked Gelfoam.

#6

Answer: B

Following a tooth extraction, there is often a protective clot overlying the site of extraction. If there is premature loss of the clot, the underlying bone becomes exposed causing severe pain. Dry sockets will usually present a few days after extraction, and patients are non-toxic appearing. The extraction site is usually unimpressive with visualization of an exposed socket. The socket can be irrigated and packed with gelfoam or eugenol for pain relief. Patients can develop fever, leukocytosis. The surrounding teeth and bone may be sensitive to palpation in settings of osteomyelitis but not with an isolated dry socket.

- *Roberts and Hedges' Clinical Procedures in Emergency Medicine. 6th edition. 2013. Chapter: 64 Emergency Dental Procedures. 1355-1356.*

#7

A 57 year old male presents complaining of neck swelling, drooling and with pain and swelling of his tongue. Which of the following would support a diagnosis of Ludwig's angina?

A. Soft tissue X-rays showing swelling, airway narrowing and a gas collection

B. Ultrasound identifying abscesses and edema

C. Gram Stain and culture displaying mixed aerobic-anaerobic bacteria

D. Complaints of dysphagia, odynophagia, drooling, neck pain and swelling, dysphonia and restricted neck movement

E. All the above

#7

Answer: E

Ludwig's angina is a progressive infection of the floor of the mouth and neck that begins in the submandibular space. Typically the nidus of infection is odontogenic. Physical exam may reveal elevation of the tongue, a woody consistency to the floor of the mouth, oral edema, anterior neck swelling, and pain. Patients can have rapid progression of airway obstruction and require emergent fibreoptic guided oral or nasotracheal intubation. IV antibiotics covering gram-positive, gram-negative, and anaerobic organisms are required in addition to head and neck surgical consult.

- *Rosen's Emergency Medicine- Concepts and Clinical Practice. 8th edition. 2013. Chapter 75: Upper Respiratory Tract Infections. 972-974.*

#8

Which of the following are the TWO most common causes of otitis externa, an acute inflammation or infection of the external ear canal.

(Choose two answers.)

A. Pseudomonas

B. Staphylococcus aureus

C. Staphylococcus epidermidis

D. Enterobacter

E. Proteus

#8

Answer: A and B

The most common bacterial pathogens are Pseudomonas, followed by Staph aureus. Staph epidermidis, Enterobacter, Proteus, and Klebsiella are less common pathogens.

- *Rosen's Emergency Medicine- Concepts and Clinical Practice. 8th edition. 2013. Chapter 72: Otolaryngology. 935-936.*

#9

Regarding mastoiditis, which of the following statements is FALSE?

A. Mastoiditis is considered a suppurative complication of acute otitis media.

B. It predominantly affects older children with 50% of cases seen in children > 3 years of age.

C. Mastoiditis is a spectrum of disease ranging from infectious inflammation of mastoid air cells to abscess development and subsequent spread to contiguous areas.

D. Most common bacterial pathogens are Strep pneumoniae, Strep pyogenes, Staph aureus, and pseudomonas.

E. CT scan may demonstrate the osteitis and abscess formation.

#9

Answer: B

Mastoiditis predominantly affects younger children with 50% of cases seen in children < 3 years of age.

- *Rosen's Emergency Medicine- Concepts and Clinical Practice. 8th edition. 2013. Chapter 72: Otolaryngology. 936-937.*

#10

You are seeing a patient with a history of sinusitis who now requests a CT scan of his sinuses. When is imaging indicated in the presentation of acute sinusitis?

(Choose four answers.)

A. If you suspect an orbital complication – orbital cellulitis, orbital abscess, or subperiosteal abscess

B. If you suspect an intracranial complication - meningitis, encephalitis, subdural abscess, osteomyelitis (Pott's puffy tumor), or cavernous sinus thrombosis

C. If the symptoms have been going on longer than 28 days despite symptomatic treatment, followed by antibiotic treatment

D. When plain radiographs demonstrate an air-fluid level

E. If the patient is immunocompromised and you suspect invasive rhinosinusitis (Mucor)

#10

Answer: A, B, C, and E

CT is the examination of choice in the evaluation of chronic sinus disease when there is a concern for a complication based on history and physical. Indications for imaging in sinusitis include:

1. Suspicion for intracranial extension causing meningitis, encephalitis, sagittal sinus thrombosis, or subdural abscess
2. Suspicion for orbital extension, causing orbital cellulitis, subperiosteal abscess, cavernous sinus thrombosis, bony invasion causing osteomyelitis or Potts Puffy tumor
3. History of immunocompromised state in patient
4. If the history is not typical of acute sinusitis
5. If the diagnosis of sinusitis is not clear from the clinical presentation and it must be ruled out from other differential diagnoses.

MRI is reserved for the evaluation of any complications of sinus infections, particularly suspected intracranial extension. Plain radiography is generally obsolete in the evaluation of sinusitis, since there are high false negative rates due to imaging limitations.

- *Rosen's Emergency Medicine - Concepts and Clinical Practice. 8th edition. 2013. Chapter 75: Upper Respiratory Tract Infections. 975-977.*

#11

A 25-year-old man presents to the emergency department with a toothache. He has been taking 12 grams of acetaminophen daily for the pain. He also drinks 3 beers daily. The patient does not have any abdominal complaints and only complains of dull tooth pain along his 2nd right upper molar. His serum acetaminophen concentration 8 hours after the most recent dose is undetectable. His serum alanine aminotransferase concentration is 75 IU per liter, his serum bilirubin concentration is 1.2 mg per deciliter (20.5 μmol per liter), and his international normalized ratio (INR) is 1.1. When you contact the poison control center they recommend treatment with N-acetylcysteine (NAC). While administering the NAC, the patient begins to complain of facial flushing. Which of the following is recommended for this side effect?

A. Subcutaneous epinephrine

B. No treatment

C. Diphenhydramine

D. Corticosteroids

E. Bronchodilators

#11

Answer: B

You thought this section was only on ENT! Well, patient with oral complaints can require a tox work up sometimes!

According to the recommendations for adverse reactions during NAC therapy, no treatment is necessary for isolated flushing. If patients develop urticaria then diphenhydramine can help relieve symptoms. Patients with angioedema, bronchospasm, or hypotension should receive benadryl, corticosteroids, and bronchodilators along with cessation of the NAC. The NAC infusion should then be started at a slower rate 1 hour after administration of medical therapy. Curiously, epinephrine is not recommended although it can be used in patients with severe progressive symptoms.

The most commonly reported adverse effects of intravenous acetylcysteine are anaphylactoid reactions, including rash, pruritus, angioedema, bronchospasm, tachycardia, and hypotension. Kerr et al. reported that approximately 15% of patients who were treated with intravenous acetylcysteine had an anaphylactoid reaction within 2 hours after the initial infusion and that increasing the infusion time from 15 to 60 minutes did not alter the rate of adverse events. Other common adverse effects included vomiting and flushing.

- *Heard KJ. Acetylcysteine for acetaminophen poisoning. N Engl J Med. 2008; 359(3): 285-92.*

#12

You are seeing a 31 year old male with a mandibular dislocation. Which of the following is the most common types of mandibular dislocations?

A. Anterior

B. Posterior

C. Superior

D. Lateral

#12

Answer: A

The mandible can dislocate in the anterior, posterior, lateral, or superior position. Description of the dislocation is based on the location of the condyle in comparison to the temporal articular groove.

- Anterior dislocations are the most common and result in displacement of the condyle anterior to the articular eminence of the temporal bone.
- Posterior dislocations typically occur secondary to a direct mandibular trauma. The mandibular condyle is pushed posteriorly toward the mastoid. Injury to the external auditory canal from the condylar head may occur from this type of injury.
- Superior dislocations occur from a direct trauma with an opened mouth. The angle of the mandible in this position results in upward migration of the condylar head and can result in facial nerve palsy.
- Lateral dislocations are usually associated with mandibular fractures. The condylar head migrates laterally and superiorly and can often be palpated in the temporal space.

Reference:

- *Roberts and Hedges' Clinical Procedures in Emergency Medicine. 6th edition. 2013. Chapter 63: Otolaryngologic Procedures. 1337-1338.*

#13

You are seeing a patient in whom you suspect malignant otitis externa. True statements about this disease process include all of the following EXCEPT:

A. Most frequently, the disease occurs in diabetic and immunocompromised patients and involves bacterial spread to the cartilage of the external ear with resulting pain and edema.

B. It may be accompanied by fever and systemic manifestations of infection.

C. Diabetic ketoacidosis frequently accompanies this diagnosis in patients who have underlying diabetes.

D. Outpatient antibiotic treatment is indicated and sufficient if coverage for pseudomonas is assured.

E. Most patients with otitis externa improve within 48-72 hours of antibiotic administration.

#13

Answer: D

Malignant otitis externa is a significant complication of acute otitis externa. Most frequently, the disease occurs in diabetic and immunocompromised patients and involves bacterial spread to the cartilage of the external ear with resulting pain and edema. It may be accompanied by a fever and systemic manifestations of infection. Treatment requires parenteral antibiotics with coverage for Pseudomonas species, in addition to local care. These patients require specialty consultation and hospitalization. The infection can spread to the pinna, resulting in a chondritis, particularly in patients with newly pierced ears. Most patients with simple otitis externa improve within 48-72 hours of antibiotic administration. Failure to improve within 2-3 days should call the diagnosis into question and prompt reevaluation. Surgical intervention is sometimes necessary for chronic otitis externa.

- *Rosen's Emergency Medicine - Concepts and Clinical Practice. 8th edition. 2013. Chapter 72: Otolaryngology. 935-936.*

#14

A young 17 year old female presents to your emergency department with dysphagia and odynophagia. On exam there is no peritonsillar abscess, but a red, enlarged and edematous uvula without any deviation. There are no tonsillar exudates. You suspect uvulitis. True statements about uvulitis include all of the following EXCEPT:

A. Uvulitis may be associated with pharyngitis.

B. Uvulitis may be associated with epiglottitis.

C. Uvulitis is always due to an infectious etiology.

D. The differential diagnosis of uvulitis includes retropharyngeal and parapharyngeal abscesses.

E. Uvulitis is a clinical diagnosis.

#14

Answer: C

Uvulitis is a clinical diagnosis. The uvula is red and swollen and may be covered by purulent exudates. There are infectious and noninfectious causes. Group A Strep is the most common cause and occurs in the setting of pharyngitis. Haemophilus influenzae B (Hib) is the next most common bacterial cause and occurs in regions with poor vaccination rates. Hib uvulitis may occur as an isolated infection or in conjunction with pharyngitis or epiglottitis.

Non-infectious uvulitis is a result of:

1. Trauma during airway or other instrumentation (eg, intubation, orogastric tube placement, upper endoscopy, adenoidectomy)
2. Inhalation of chemical irritants (including cannabis)
3. Inhalation of steam (and presumably other sources of heated air)
4. Vasculitis (eg, Kawasaki disease)
5. Allergic reactions
6. Angioedema of the uvula
7. Hereditary angioneurotic edema, with or without C1 inhibitor deficiency
8. Angiotensin-converting enzyme inhibitor-associated with angioedema

. *Roberts and Hedges' Clinical Procedures in Emergency Medicine. 6th edition. 2013. Chapter 63: Otolaryngologic Procedures. 1340-1341.*

#15

You are seeing a patient in whom you suspect otitis externa. True statements about this disease process include all of the following EXCEPT:

A. The most common organisms reported in otitis externa are staphylococcus and streptococcus species.

B. If left untreated, the infection may invade the deeper adjacent structures and progress into malignant otitis externa.

C. The sine qua non of otitis externa is pain on gentle traction of the external ear structures.

D. By definition, cranial nerve (CN) involvement (ie, of CNs VII and IX-XII) is not associated with simple otitis externa.

E. In the case of a perforated tympanic membrane, it is critical to avoid using the otic solution, which increases the risk of aminoglycoside ototoxicity. In this setting, suspension drops are safer to use.

#15

Answer: A

The most common organism reported in otitis externa is Pseudomonas species, followed by Staphylococcus and Streptococcus species. Fungi are a less common cause of otitis externa. Once an infection becomes established, localized maceration and inflammation occur. If the process progresses to malignant otitis externa, the infection can invade the deeper underlying structures of the soft tissue and temporal bone. Malignant otitis externa is a complication seen more often in immunocompromised patients or poorly controlled diabetics.

A recent literature review concluded that the use of ciprofloxacin 0.3%/dexamethasone 0.1% otic suspension for otitis externa is safe and effective and that dexamethasone improves treatment success. Fluoroquinolones are not associated with ototoxicity, and ofloxacin is safe in cases of a perforated tympanic membrane.

- *Rosen's Emergency Medicine- Concepts and Clinical Practice. 8th edition. 2013. Chapter 72: Otolaryngology. 935-936.*

- *Wall GM, et al. Ciprofloxacin 0.3%/dexamethasone 0.1% sterile otic suspension for the topical treatment of ear infections: A Review of the Literature. Pediatr Infect Dis J. 2009 Feb; 28(2): 141-4.*

#16

You are seeing a patient in whom you suspect Strep pharyngitis. True statements about this diagnosis include all of the following EXCEPT:

A. Cough is a common symptom of GAS pharyngitis.

B. A history of orogenital contact is more consistent with gonococcal pharyngitis.

C. Headache is consistent with GAS pharyngitis.

D. Sudden onset is more consistent with GAS pharyngitis, rather than a viral etiology.

E. GAS pharyngitis is most common in the 4-7 year old age group.

#16

Answer: A

Cough is not usually associated with GAS infection. In fact, the absence of a cough is one of the Centor criteria, which include:

1. Fever
2. Anterior cervical lymphadenopathy
3. Tonsillar exudate
4. Absence of cough

Each criteria is given one point, with patients scoring 0-1 unlikely to have GAS infection and patients with a score of 4 more likely to have GAS. In adults, the positive predictive value of the Centor criteria for predicting GAS pharyngitis is around 40% if 3 criteria are met, and about 50% if 4 criteria are met. GAS infection is most common in children aged 4-7 years. Sudden onset is consistent with a GAS pharyngitis. Other upper respiratory symptoms such as coughing or rhinorrhea are more likely in viral etiologies. Suspect gonococcal pharyngitis if patients have a history of recent orogenital contact, especially in the setting of copious purulent exudates.

- *McIsaac WJ, et al. Empirical validation of guidelines for the management of pharyngitis in children and adults. JAMA. 2004; 291(13): 1587–1595.*
- *MDCalc Modified Centor http://www.mdcalc.com/modified-centor-score-for-strep-pharyngitis/*

#17

You are seeing a patient who presented with submandibular pain and a mass, and a noncontrast CT scan demonstrated a salivary stone. Which of the following statements below is FALSE?

A. Submandibular gland stones are more common than parotid duct stones.

B. One of the treatment modalities includes the administration of anticholinergic agents.

C. Most stones < 2mm pass spontaneously.

D. When sialadenitis occurs (bacterial infection due to an obstructed stone), then antistaphylococcal antibiotic should be administered.

E. Most patients with sialolithiasis present with pain and a mass.

#17

Answer: B

Salivary gland stones commonly occur in the parotid, submandibular, and sublingual salivary glands. The majority occur within the submandibular glands, most often occurring as single stone within Wharton's duct. Dehydration, anti-cholinergic medications and trauma predispose to the formation of stones. Patients commonly present with facial pain and a palpable mass over the location of the affected salivary gland. Treatment is mainly conservative with adequate hydration and warm compresses applied to the area of swelling. Other common therapies are use of tart hard candies or lemons to promote salivary flow and NSAIDs to reduce swelling and help with pain. Since anticholinergic medications are a common cause, they should be discontinued. If there is evidence of sialadenitis then antibiotics should target Staphylococcal species. Most stones smaller than 2 mm will pass spontaneously over a few days. Rarely is lithotripsy or surgical extraction required unless patients have prolonged symptoms or failed conservative therapy.

- *Rosen's Emergency Medicine- Concepts and Clinical Practice. 8th edition. 2013. Chapter 72: Otolaryngology. 939.*

#18

You are seeing a patient with an ear foreign body and you are considering using irrigation. When is this method CONTRAINDICATED?

(Choose three answers.)

A. Patients with suspected tympanic membrane perforation

B. Patient with tympanostomy tubes

C. Patients with organic foreign bodies

D. Pediatric patients

E. Elderly patients

#18

Answer: A, B, and C

Irrigation is contraindicated in patients with suspected or known tympanic membrane perforation or those with tympanostomy tubes. In addition, irrigation should not be used in those with organic foreign bodies, since water may make the object swell, and increase the difficulty of removal.

- *Roberts and Hedges' Clinical Procedures in Emergency Medicine. 6th edition. 2013. Chapter 63: Otolaryngologic Procedures. 1313.*

#19

You are seeing a patient with otitis externa. TRUE statements about this diagnosis include which of the following?

(Choose two answers.)

A. Acute otitis externa is an inflammatory condition of the ear canal, with or without infection.

B. Symptoms include ear discomfort, itchiness, discharge and impaired hearing.

C. Optimal treatment modality includes systemic antibiotics.

D. Hospitalization is required for diabetics.

E. All of the above

#19

Answer: A and B

Acute otitis externa is an inflammatory condition of the ear canal, with or without infection. It is also referred to as "swimmer's ear" and patients will complain of ear pain, discharge and pruritus. According to a Cochrane review of randomized controlled trials evaluating treatment, topical antimicrobials with steroids are sufficient for treatment. Unless there are signs of severe illness or malignant otitis externa, systemic antibiotics are not necessary. Treatment should proceed for 7-10 days with relief of symptoms beginning after 5 days of use. Patients with persisting symptoms beyond two weeks should be considered treatment failures and may require alternative therapies or surgical debridement.

- *Vivek Kaushik, Malik T, Saeed SR. Interventions for acute otitis externa. Cochrane Database Syst Rev. 2010 Jan 20; (1): CD004740.*

#20

Regarding treatment for epistaxis, which of the following is TRUE?

(Choose two answers.)

A. When chemical cautery with silver nitrate is used, the optimal way to obtain hemostasis and avoid complications is to cauterize both sides.

B. Nasal packing, with products such as Rapid Rhino, and Merocel packing may be used.

C. Patients who are successfully packed posteriorly or with bilateral anterior packs are best sent home with follow-up in 1 week for packing removal.

D. If hemostasis can not be obtained, interventional radiology can embolize the internal carotid artery or ligate it to obtain proximal control.

E. When nasal packs are in place, oral antibiotics are prescribed because of the concern for toxic shock syndrome.

#20

Answer: B and E

Chemical cautery is a possible treatment for epistaxis that is refractory to pressure and topical vasoconstrictors. Bilateral cauterization should not be used due to the risk of nasal septum perforation. For chemical cautery to be effective, there cannot be active bleeding.Anterior nasal packing is used for epistaxis that originates in Kisselbach's area and is refractory to other treatments. Absorbable packing (Surgicel, Gelfoam) or non absorbable packing (Merocel) can be used. The packs are left in place for 1-3 days with follow-up and removal by ENT specialist. Inflatable packs such as the Rapid Rhino can also be used for a greater level of hemostasis. When nasal packs are placed, topical antibiotic ointments and oral antibiotics are prescribed to decrease the theoretical risk of toxic shock syndrome. The practice of antibiotic use originated from a study of patients undergoing nasal surgery who had an incidence of toxic shock of 16.5 cases per 100,000. Due to the rarity of toxic shock syndrome, no data has shown that antibiotic use has reduced its incidence. In the rare case where no therapy can stop bleeding and the presumed source is posterior, embolization by interventional radiology or surgical ligation by ENT is required. The internal maxillary artery is the main target of embolization, not the internal carotid.

- *Rodney J. Schlosser. Clinical practice. Epistaxis. N Engl J Med. 2009 Feb 19; 360(8): 784-9. full text*

- *Williams PWA, et al. Endovascular Treatment of Epistaxis. AJNR. 2009 Oct; 30(9): 1637-45. full text*

#21

Regarding epistaxis, which of the following statements is TRUE?

(Choose two answers.)

A. 50% of epistaxis occurs in the anterior nasal septum, and 50% occur posteriorly.

B. Posterior nasal bleeds are more common in children.

C. The association between hypertension and epistaxis is evidence-based, and thus, blood pressure should be acutely lowered if it is elevated in a patient who presents with epistaxis.

D. Recurrent unilateral epistaxis that does not respond to the simple conservative measures should raise suspicion for neoplasm.

E. Most anterior nosebleeds are self-limited and do not require medical treatment.

#21

Answer: D and E

More than 90% of episodes of epistaxis occur along the anterior nasal septum at Kiesselbach's plexus. Although commonly thought of as a venous plexus, it is actually an arterial plexus resulting from convergence of the superior labial branch of the facial artery, the terminal branches of the sphenopalatine artery and from the internal carotid artery through the anterior and posterior ethmoidal arteries. The remaining 10% of nosebleeds will occur posteriorly from the sphenopalatine branch of the internal maxillary artery.

Although patients with epistaxis may have hypertension, the severity of hypertension is not associated with the severity of bleeding. Recurrent unilateral epistaxis that does not respond to the simple conservative measures should raise suspicion for neoplasm. Most anterior nosebleeds are self-limited and do not require medical treatment and respond to pressure applied to the anterior nose for 15 minutes.

- *Rodney J. Schlosser. Clinical practice. Epistaxis. N Engl J Med. 2009 Feb 19; 360(8): 784-9. full text*
- *Knopfholz J, et al. Association between epistaxis and hypertension: a one year follow-up after an index episode of nose bleeding in hypertensive patients. Int J Cardiol. 2009 May 29; 134(3): e107-9.*

#22

Regarding local causes of dental pain, which of the following statements is TRUE?

A. Gingivitis refers to non-specific inflammation of the gums and can present with pain, bleeding, or localized swelling.

B. Pericoronitis is inflammation of the gingival tissue over a previously extracted tooth.

C. Both of the above

D. Neither of the above

#22

Answer: A

Gingivitis refers to non-specific inflammation of the gums, and patients may present to the ED with pain, bleeding, or localized swelling of the gingiva. It can result from a buildup of dental bacterial plaque, local trauma, systemic disease, or a variety of medications. In the majority of cases, saline rinses and topical or systemic analgesia are sufficient. With significant inflammation or local trauma, an oral antibiotic may also be necessary.

Pericoronitis is an inflammation of the gingival tissue overlying an erupting tooth, rather than over an extracted tooth. This tissue is referred to as the operculum, and food and debris can easily become impacted, resulting in both inflammation and infection. ED management consists of local irrigation and removal of the debris trapped under the operculum, followed by saline mouth rinses, analgesia, NSAIDS, and oral antibiotics. Penicillin or clindamycin provides adequate coverage for dental flora. A soft diet, good oral hygiene and referral for definitive care with a general dentist is appropriate.

- *Rosen's Emergency Medicine - Concepts and Clinical Practice. 8th edition. 2013. Chapter: 70: Oral Medicine. 899-901.*

#23

Regarding local causes of dental pain, which of the following statements is TRUE?

A. Acute necrotizing ulcerative gingivitis (ANUG) results from an overgrowth of normal oral flora, and it is treated with antibiotics and improved local hygiene.

B. A periapical abscess with local subperiosteal spread will be visible as a swelling of the gingival adjacent to the involved tooth and will be tender and fluctuant on palpation.

C. Both of the above

D. Neither of the above

#23

Answer: C

ANUG is an invasive infection of the gingiva and results from an overgrowth of normal oral flora, and is more common in the immunosuppressed or diabetic. The condition is painful, and patients often have systemic manifestations of fever with ulcerative gingival margins and grey membranes and exudates. Complications result from tracking of the bacteria in areas of poor dentition or prior exposed alveolar bone and can result in osteomyelitis or abscesses. Pus may track from the apex of the root to the underlying alveolar bone, and a periapical abscess forms.

Mouthwash rinses and antibiotics (penicillin VK 250 mg four times a day or doxycycline 100 mg twice daily for 10 days) are usually effective unless the patient has further oral complications. Surgical debridement is rarely necessary.

- *Rosen's Emergency Medicine- Concepts and Clinical Practice. 8th edition. 2013. Chapter: 70: Oral Medicine. 899-901.*

#24

Regarding Ludwig's angina, which of the following is TRUE?

(Choose three answers.)

A. Ludwig's is a progressive cellulitis of the floor of the mouth, typically from an infected or recently extracted lower second or third molar.

B. Infections are typically monomicrobial with staphylococcus.

C. Symptoms include dysphagia, voice changes, and drooling.

D. The first priority is administration of antibiotics.

E. With early treatment, mortality is < 10%.

#24

Answer: A, C, and E

Ludwig's angina is a polymicrobial infection (staphylococcus, streptococcus, bacteroides species, and anaerobes) involving the floor of the mouth. The cellulitis commonly spreads from a dental source and progresses to the sublingual and submandibular space. The greatest and first priority is early airway control, preferably via fiberoptic assist with preparation for cricothyrotomy or surgical tracheostomy. IV antibiotics should be started early. With early treatment, mortality is < 10%.

- *Rosen's Emergency Medicine - Concepts and Clinical Practice. 8th edition. 2013. Chapter 75: Upper Respiratory Tract Infections. 972-974.*

#25

Which of the following is the most important factor in predicting success rate of a reimplanted tooth?

A. Age of the patient

B. Mechanism of injury

C. Thorough cleaning of the tooth and root prior to reimplantation

D. Time to reimplantation

#25

Answer: D

In permanent teeth avulsion, reimplantation should be undertaken as soon as possible. The success rate of reimplantation is directly related to the time the tooth has been out of the socket. Care should be applied to the periodontal ligament fibers since preservation increases the chance of re-implantation success. Teeth should be handled by the crown and aggressive irrigation should be avoided. Primary teeth should not be reimplanted. A balanced pH liquid such as Hank's solution, the patient's own saliva, or milk are all options for preventing cell death.

- *Roberts and Hedges' Clinical Procedures in Emergency Medicine. 6th edition. 2013. Chapter 64: Emergency Dental Procedures. 1350.*

#26

Which of the following is the ideal position for reduction of a mandibular dislocation?

A. The patient should be in a standing position at eye level with the examiner.

B. The patient should be supine on a stretcher with the examiner at the head of the bed.

C. The patient should be supine on a stretcher with the examiner at the right side of the bed.

D. The patient may be in the seated position with a firm surface behind his or her head facing the examiner.

#26

Answer: D

IV analgesia is usually sufficient for pain control prior to reduction. Procedural sedation is rarely necessary. Local analgesia with 2% lidocaine placed into the joint space, which can be felt as a depression just anterior to the tragus, can also aid in reduction. The patient should be seated facing the examiner, with his or her head resting against a firm surface. The examiner should stand and place both gloved thumbs along the occlusal surfaces of the mandibular molars. The patient should try to open the jaw as far as possible and relax the jaw muscles. The examiner should place slow, steady downward and backward pressure to dislodge the mandible. Once successfully reduced, most patients can be discharged home with OMFS follow-up, instructions for a soft diet, and to avoid opening the mouth wide. In cases of an associated fracture, OMFS consultation is necessary. You can also attempt standing behind the patient while the patient is sitting to obtain good leverage using a similar downward and backward pressure.

. *Roberts and Hedges' Clinical Procedures in Emergency Medicine. 6th edition. 2013. Chapter 63: Otolaryngologic Procedures. 1337-1338.*

#27

Tripod fractures involve which bones?

A. Lateral orbit, zygoma, and the maxilla

B. Medial orbit, nasal bones, and the maxilla

C. Orbital floor, nasal bones, and the maxilla

D. Zygoma, medial orbit, and lateral orbit

E. None of the above

#27

Answer: A

Tripod fractures (zygomaticomaxillary fractures) involve:

1. The lateral orbit
2. The zygoma
3. The maxilla

The fracture requires operative repair because they are unstable and will produce a sunken appearance to the face.

- *Rosen's Emergency Medicine- Concepts and Clinical Practice. 8th edition. 2013. Chapter 42: Facial Trauma. 374.*

#28

True or False: A patient who has a blowout fracture of the orbital floor and has inferior rectus entrapment requires an IMMEDIATE surgical repair.

A. True

B. False

#28

Answer: B

A complication of orbital floor fractures is inferior rectus muscle entrapment. There will be limitation of upward gaze on exam. Since soft tissue edema often contributes to the limitation of upward gaze, surgical repair is indicated for persistent enophthalmos or diplopia. The surgery may be performed up to a week after the injury. In children the surgery may be more emergent due to the hinging and trap-door like entrapment that prevents release of the inferior rectus.

- *Rosen's Emergency Medicine- Concepts and Clinical Practice. 8th edition. 2013. Chapter 42: Facial Trauma. 372.*

#29

True or False: After replantation of an avulsed tooth, it can take several weeks to assess the final success of reimplantation.

A. True

B. False

#29

Answer: A

True. It takes several weeks to determine the success of a replanted tooth. The greater the time to replantation, the greater the rate of failure. The success rate decreases significantly for every minute the tooth is not replanted.

- *Rosen's Emergency Medicine- Concepts and Clinical Practice. 8th edition. 2013. Chapter 70: Oral Medicine. 903-904.*

#30

You are working in an ED that sees both adults and children. A 55 year old grandfather who has a right neck mass brings in his 3 year old grandson who has a left neck mass. Which of the following are risk factors for ENT malignancies in both of these patients?

A. Alcohol and tobacco

B. Viruses such as herpes

C. Sunlight

D. Genetics

E. Inhalation exposures

F. All of the above

#30

Answer: E

In addition to all of the above listed factors, diet and exposure to dust are also considered risk factors. Children and young adults are more likely to have benign disorders, such as thyroglossal or branchial cleft cysts. In general, 80% of nonthyroidal neck masses in adults are neoplastic; of which 80% are malignant. In children, however, more than 80% of neck masses are benign, and this is often referred to as the rule of 80.

. *Connolly, AA, MacKenzie, K. Paediatric Neck Masses – a diagnostic dilemma. J Laryngol Otol. 1997 Jun;111(6): 541-5.*

ENVIRONMENTAL

#1

Regarding acute radiation injury, which of the following statements is FALSE?

A. Similar to thermal burns, acute radiation injury to the skin causes immediate desquamation and blistering.

B. Larger total body doses correlate with increasing acuity of symptoms and decreasing time interval to onset.

C. Hospital personnel caring for victims of radiation exposure should wear a radiation detector to determine the whole body dose accumulated during patient contact.

D. Life-threatening injuries take precedence over assessment of radiation contamination assessment.

E. Removal of all clothing eliminates 80 to 90% of external contamination.

#1

Answer: A

Acute radiation injury to the skin and underlying structures causes changes that clinically resemble thermal burns, with desquamation and blistering. Unlike thermal burns, these signs develop after a period of at least 48 to 72 hours (up to 2 weeks) after contact. Delayed skin effects include carcinogenesis, vascular insufficiency, and chronic non-healing ulcers.

- *Rosen's Emergency Medicine - Concepts and Clinical Practice. 8th edition. 2013. Chapter 146: Radiation Injuries. 1949-1950.*

#2

Regarding the management and treatment of radiation injuries, which of the following statements is FALSE?

A. Prussian blue should be administered as soon as cesium or thallium has been identified as the radionuclide in question.

B. Potassium iodine should be administered if plutonium exposure is suspected.

C. Lymphocyte count is routinely used to aid in disposition and management of radiation injuries, as prognosis is directly tied to the 48 hour lymphocyte count which is dose dependent.

D. Onset of prodromal acute radiation sickness (ARS) symptoms (anorexia, nausea, vomiting, and diarrhea) less than 30 minutes after exposure indicates a total body dose greater than 600 rads (mortality 100% within 30 days without medical support).

E. Onset of prodromal ARS symptoms greater than 24 hours after exposure indicates a dose less than 70 rads.

#2

Answer: B

Potassium iodine (KI) should only be administered to only those in whom exposure to Iodine-131 is likely. KI works by competitively preventing the incorporation of radioactive iodine by the thyroid gland. It will protect the thyroid from increased risk for cancer but will not mitigate any other forms of acute or long-term radiation effects. Calcium and Zinc DTPA can be given for suspected plutonium exposure.

In general the sooner the onset of emesis, the greater the radiation exposure. Decrease in the absolute lymphocyte count within 48hrs is the best predictor of severity of radiation exposure.

- *Rosen's Emergency Medicine - Concepts and Clinical Practice. 8th edition. 2013. Chapter 146: Radiation Injuries. 1951-1952.*

#3

Regarding decompression sickness (DCS), which of the following statements is FALSE?

A. Patients with suspected DCS should receive 100% oxygen by nonrebreather face mask or endotracheal tube if necessary to ensure and intact airway.

B. Recompression with hyperbaric oxygen (HBO) should occur as soon as possible, with transfer to a recompression center if necessary.

C. Clinicians unfamiliar with treatment of underwater diving injuries should consult a diving or hyperbaric medicine specialist or the Divers Alert Network (DAN) (919-684-8111).

D. DCS can be delayed in onset, improve spontaneously and then relapse, or occur after traveling from remote locations.

E. An arterial gas embolism will most often embolize to the lungs.

#3

Answer: E

Gas from an arterial gas embolism most prominently involves the brain, and is called Cerebral Arterial Gas Embolism (CAGE). A diver with CAGE will develop symptoms during ascent or immediately on surfacing. Symptoms include altered level of consciousness, hemiplegia, hemiparesis, seizure, or other cerebral dysfunction. Any neurologic symptom in the setting of pulmonary barotrauma should be thought to be secondary to CAGE.

- *Rosen's Emergency Medicine - Concepts and Clinical Practice. 8th edition. 2013. Chapter 143: SCUBA Diving and Dysbarism. 1920-1922.*

#4

You suspect that a young 25 year old male has acute mountain sickness (AMS). He presents with headache, nausea, anorexia, malaise, dry mucus membranes and shortness of breath, 12 hours after arriving to the ski resort. Arterial blood gas demonstrates hypoxia and hypocapnia, with respiratory alkalosis. Which of the following statements is FALSE about AMS?

A. Descent is the most effective treatment for AMS.

B. Acetazolamide relieves symptoms, improves arterial oxygenation, and prevents further impairment of gas exchange.

C. Dexamethasone PO, IV, or IM may also be effective for the treatment of AMS.

D. Diuretics should be administered to this patient.

E. CPAP or BiPAP, or endotracheal ventilation may be necessary for patients with respiratory failure.

#4

Answer: D

Patients with vomiting should be given antiemetics and hydrated with intravenous saline. Diuretics are not helpful and may be harmful in patients with underlying dehydration. In fact, most patients will be dehydrated and require fluids. All of the other statements are true.

- *Rosen's Emergency Medicine - Concepts and Clinical Practice. 8th edition. 2013. Chapter 144: High-Altitude Medicine. 1928-1933.*

#5

You are treating a patient with suspected heatstroke. All of the following statements about heat-related illnesses are true, EXCEPT:

A. The patient should be immersed or cooled with ice, prior to all other interventions.

B. Cooling is continued only until the temperature drops to 38.5-39 °C to avoid overshoot hypothermia.

C. Shivering may be treated with intravenous benzodiazepines. Avoid neuroleptics like chlorpromazine due to anticholinergic properties that interfere with sweating.

D. Seizure activity is best treated with diazepam or thiopental, as phenytoin is ineffective in this setting.

E. In contrast to neuroleptic malignant syndrome, patients with heatstroke have muscular rigidity that does not respond to dantrolene.

#5

Answer: A

The cornerstone of heat stroke therapy is rapid cooling. However, immersing or covering the patient in ice is not recommended because skin cooling causes both vasoconstriction and shivering and may increase the core temperature. Immersion also complicates the resuscitation. Although the fastest cooling rates have been reported with peritoneal and thoracic lavage, the combination of evaporative cooling and iced gastric lavage is just as effective and more practical. Evaporation is maximized without inducing shivering by keeping the patient wet with lukewarm water or wet towels and blowing air over him or her with a fan. Cooling blankets may be effective for patients with mild heat stroke.

- *Rosen's Emergency Medicine - Concepts and Clinical Practice. 8th edition. 2013. Chapter 141: Heat Illness. 1904-1933.*

#6

All of the following statements about heatstroke are true, EXCEPT:

A. Although in heatstroke the core temperature is elevated above 40.5 ºC, significant cooling may occur in the prehospital, and the first temperature obtained in the ED may not represent the maximum.

B. Victims of classic heatstroke are often prescribed medications (e.g., diuretics, antihypertensives, neuroleptics, and anticholinergics) that impair the ability to tolerate heat stress.

C. In contrast to patients with classic heatstroke, patients with exertional heatstroke are usually young and healthy people, whose normal heat-dispelling mechanisms are overwhelmed by endogenous heat production.

D. One effective treatment modality is to use acetaminophen or aspirin.

E. Hepatic damage is common in heatstroke and the diagnosis should be questioned if transaminases are normal.

#6

Answer: D

Aspirin and other antipyretics block the action of the pyrogen at hypothalamic receptor sites through inhibition of prostaglandin synthesis. Antipyretics are not effective against and should not be used to control environmental hyperthermia (heat stroke). In fact, aspirin can exacerbate the acid-base disturbances that commonly occur in the setting of heat stroke.

- *Rosen's Emergency Medicine - Concepts and Clinical Practice. 8th edition. 2013. Chapter 141: Heat Illness. 1903-1904.*

#7

You are treating a patient with an electrical injury and are determining whether the patient can go home. All of the following are indications for cardiac monitoring EXCEPT:

A. Dysrhythmia observed in the emergency department

B. Hypoxia

C. Cardiac arrest

D. Age > 65

E. Chest pain

#7

Answer: D

Cardiac arrest, loss of consciousness, abnormal ECG, arrhythmias observed in the prehospital or emergency department setting, suspicion of conductive injury, hypoxia, and chest pain are all indications for cardiac monitoring after an electrical injury.

- *Rosen's Emergency Medicine - Concepts and Clinical Practice. 8th edition. 2013. Chapter 142: Electrical and Lightning Injuries. 1913-1914.*

#8

You are with a fellow mountain climber, and you are both on a high altitude trek. He begins to complain of nausea, headache, insomnia, dizziness, and dyspnea on exertion after 12 hours of being at this altitude. Which of the following would be appropriate management options?

A. Descend 500 m or more.

B. If descent is impossible, then use a portable hyperbaric chamber.

C. If descent is impossible, administer oxygen at 1-2 L/min.

D. If descent and additional oxygen are not possibilities, then consider acetazolamide 250mg PO BID plus dexamethasone 4 mg PO every 6h until symptoms resolve.

E. All of the above

#8

Answer: E

These are symptoms of moderate acute mountain sickness. Descent of 500m or more is the primary treatment. If descent is not possible, then using a portable hyperbaric chamber or administering oxygen are options. If neither of these is possible, then administration of acetazolamide 250 mg PO BID and dexamethasone 8 mg initially followed by 4 mg PO Q6hrs are appropriate management options.

- *Rosen's Emergency Medicine - Concepts and Clinical Practice. 8th edition. 2013. Chapter 144: High-Altitude Medicine. 1928-1933.*

#9

Which of the following does NOT increase the risk of developing decompression sickness (DCS)?

A. Rapid descent

B. Repetitive dives

C. Subsequent altitude exposure

D. Rapid ascent

E. None of the above

#9

Answer: A

Rapid ascent, repetitive dives, and subsequent altitude exposure are all risk factors for developing DCS after a dive.

- *Rosen's Emergency Medicine - Concepts and Clinical Practice. 8th edition. 2013. Chapter 143: SCUBA Diving and Dysbarism. 1921-1922*

#10

Decompression sickness (DCS) is classified according to the organs affected. Type I DCS involves the joints, extremities, and skin. Type II DCS includes all of the following EXCEPT:

A. Neurological DCS – spinal cord paresis in compressed air sport divers

B. Vestibular DCS – "staggers"

C. Cardiopulmonary DCS – the "chokes"

D. Lymphatic obstruction

#10

Answer: D

Type I DCS is traditionally pain - musculoskeletal system, skin, and lymphatic vessels. Lymphatic obstruction can cause lymphedema, and it is a form of Type I DCS ("pain only" DCS).

Type II DCS is known as "serious DCS" and includes neurological, vestibular, and cardiopulmonary DCS. Regardless of the distinction, all types of decompression illness require recompression.

- *Rosen's Emergency Medicine - Concepts and Clinical Practice. 8th edition. 2013. Chapter 143: SCUBA Diving and Dysbarism. 1921.*

#11

Which of the following statements about underwater and diving injuries is FALSE?

A. Decompression sickness (DCS) and cerebral air embolism can be delayed in onset.

B. DCS should be considered in any patient with neurological symptoms after underwater diving.

C. Barotrauma can not occur at shallow depths or breath-holding dives.

D. It is important to consult a diving or hyperbaric medicine specialist or the Divers Alert Network for advice when the diagnosis is not clear.

#11

Answer: C

Barotrauma can occur at shallow depths, and even after breath-holding dives. The most common form of barotrauma is a middle ear "squeeze". During descent, air within the middle ear is contracting as the pressure increases, causing inward movement of the tympanic membrane. If the pressure in the middle ear is not equalized, the tympanic membrane can be injured. The diver with otic barotrauma may present with a history of difficulty clearing the affected ear, pain, a conductive hearing loss, and sometimes vertigo.

- *Rosen's Emergency Medicine - Concepts and Clinical Practice. 8th edition. 2013. Chapter 143: SCUBA Diving and Dysbarism. 1918-1922.*

#12

The most common cause of death after a lightning injury is:

A. Burns

B. Renal failure from myoglobinuria

C. Stroke

D. Cardiopulmonary arrest

E. Associated trauma

#12

Answer: D

The most common cause of death after a lightning injury is cardiopulmonary arrest. The lightning acts as a massive direct countershock which depolarizes the entire myocardium and causes asystole. Primary respiratory arrest as a result of lightning-induced paralysis of the medullary center can also result. The critical factor in determining mortality appears to be the duration of apnea, rather than the duration of asystole.

- *Rosen's Emergency Medicine - Concepts and Clinical Practice. 8th edition. 2013. Chapter 142: Electrical and Lightning Injuries. 1911-1914.*

#13

You are resuscitating an apparent victim of a lightning strike. The patient has return of spontaneous circulation, but his pupils are fixed and dilated. You should:

A. Terminate the resuscitation immediately

B. Continue resuscitation for a longer time period than if he had just been brought in as a simple cardiopulmonary arrest

C. Begin transfusing blood immediately, as the most likely cause of his fixed and dilated pupils is due to hypovolemia.

D. None of the above

#13

Answer: B

Due to the autonomic dysfunction associated with keraunoparalysis (fixed and dilated pupils; lower extremity cyanosis and paralysis from vasospasm) that can occur after electrical injuries, and classically with high voltage lightning injuries, resuscitation should continue for a prolonged period of time despite fixed and dilated pupils. Prognostication for return of neurologic activity is difficult early in the resuscitation. The patient should receive aggressive care especially since there was return of spontaneous circulation.

- *Rosen's Emergency Medicine - Concepts and Clinical Practice. 8th edition. 2013. Chapter 142: Electrical and Lightning Injuries. 1912-1914.*

#14

True statements about hypothermia, include all of the following EXCEPT:

A. Hypothermia is defined as a core temperature below 35°C (95°F) and can be further classified by severity.

B. In response to a cold stress, the hypothalamus attempts to stimulate heat production through shivering and increased thyroid, catecholamine, and adrenal activity.

C. In addition to hypothermia from environmental exposure, many medical conditions can result in hypothermia, including hypothyroidism, adrenal insufficiency, sepsis, neuromuscular disease, malnutrition, thiamine deficiency, hypoglycemia, carbon monoxide intoxication, and ethanol abuse.

D. Rough handling of the moderate or severe hypothermic patient can precipitate arrhythmias, including ventricular fibrillation, that are often unresponsive to defibrillation and medications.

E. Hypothermic patients in cardiac arrest should not be defibrillated because defibrillation can precipitate further arrhythmias.

#14

Answer: E

Ventricular arrhythmias and asystole may be refractory to conventional therapy until the patient has been rewarmed. Hypothermic patients in cardiac arrest should receive initial defibrillation and pharmacologic therapy as indicated. If initial attempts are unsuccessful, CPR and aggressive rewarming must be promptly initiated. Further efforts at defibrillation and pharmacologic therapy should be attempted again after the core temperature reaches 30 to 32°C (86 to 90°F). Bradycardia may be physiologic in severe hypothermia, and cardiac pacing generally is NOT required unless the bradycardia persists despite rewarming to 32 to 35°C (90 to 95°F).

- *Rosen's Emergency Medicine - Concepts and Clinical Practice. 8th edition. 2013. Chapter 140: Accidental Hypothermia. 1888-1891.*

#15

Of the following methods of rewarming, which is the most rapid?

A. Warmed IV fluids

B. Warmed air

C. Warmed blankets

D. Peritoneal lavage

E. Cardiopulmonary bypass

#15

Answer: E

In general, passive external rewarming is ideal for previously healthy adults with mild hypothermia. A patient who is only mildly hypothermic should be covered with dry insulating materials in a warm environment and as thermoregulatory mechanisms generate heat and warm the body. This method depends on innate thermogenesis mechanisms, and it will therefore not be effective if the patient is colder than 86°F (30°C). Passive external rewarming is reported to raise the core temperature 0.5-4 degrees Celsius/hour.

Active external rewarming is the direct application of heat to the body and may be accomplished by delivering exogenous heat externally or to the core. This includes methods such as heating pads, warm blankets, hot water bottles, radiant heat sources, warm water immersion, and forced air rewarming. Active external rewarming is reported to increase the core temperature 1-4 degrees Celsius/hour.

Active core rewarming is the direct application of heat to the core of the body through heated inhalation, gastric lavage, heated infusion, peritoneal lavage, hemodialysis, and extracorporeal warming. Cardiopulmonary bypass should be considered in unstable hypothermic patients in cardiac arrest, and it has been reported to raise the core temperature 9.5 degrees Celsius/hour. Cardiopulmonary bypass requires anticoagulation and may worsen the coagulopathy of hypothermia.

. *Rosen's Emergency Medicine - Concepts and Clinical Practice. 8th edition. 2013. Chapter 140: Accidental Hypothermia. 1891-1894.*

#16

A swimmer who was initially hypothermic in the field is brought in with warm blankets wrapped around his extremities but still wearing his wet shirt and shorts. He is initially normothermic on arrival but then 1 hour later is hypothermic again. This is an example of:

A. Heat exhaustion

B. Vasoconstriction

C. Hypothyroidism

D. Afterdrop

E. Rhabdomyolysis

#16

Answer: D

When applying external heat to the body, the return of pooled, cool blood from the previously vasoconstricted extremities may further lower the core temperature, causing after-drop and possibly causing dysrhythmias. Rewarming of the trunk first may prevent this problem by allowing warm blood to perfuse the distally constricted cold extremities. Core temperature after-drop is also more common in dehydrated patients and in patients who have frostbitten extremities.

- *Rosen's Emergency Medicine - Concepts and Clinical Practice. 8th edition. 2013. Chapter 140: Accidental Hypothermia. 1885.*

#17

Which of the following is TRUE about initial defibrillation in a severely hypothermic patient with ventricular fibrillation?

A. There is no need to defibrillate a hypothermic patient.

B. Defibrillation should be with half the joules as for a normothermic patient.

C. Defibrillation should be with twice the joules as for a normothermic patient.

D. Only pharmacologic methods should be used.

E. Defibrillation should be exactly the same as for a normothermic patient.

#17

Answer: E

If the hypothermic patient has ventricular fibrillation, biphasic defibrillation should be attempted with 2 watts/sec/kg up to 200 watt sec (Joules). The energy requirement for defibrillation does not increase with hypothermia. If the attempt is unsuccessful in a patient whose core temperature is less than 32 °C, defibrillation should not be attempted again until warming starts and the core temperature reaches 32 °C. Attempts should be repeated after every 1 °C rise in core temperature. Defibrillation should not be attempted if the patient has asystole.

- *Rosen's Emergency Medicine - Concepts and Clinical Practice. 8th edition. 2013. Chapter 140: Accidental Hypothermia. 1890.*

#18

There is an adage that "no one is dead until he is warm and dead." However, in a hypothermic patient who has no signs of life, which of the following would be highly predictive of death and suggest that resuscitation efforts are futile?

A. Dilated pupils

B. Potassium > 10.0

C. Sodium less than 130

D. Total CPK > 1000

E. pH of 7.0

F. No respirations for 15 seconds

#18

Answer: B

Adequate time (at least 3 minutes) must be allowed to determine if the patient has respirations or a heartbeat. However, clearly, some individuals are dead or will not survive. Contraindications to CPR are:

1. A non-compressible chest
2. Ice formation of the airway
3. Decapitation or other injury incompatible with life.

Victims of non-immersion hypothermic cardiac arrest with a potassium > 9 or a pH < 6.5 are not expected to survive, and a potassium > 10 is highly predictive of death. The hyperkalemia is caused by massive cell lysis.

- *Rosen's Emergency Medicine - Concepts and Clinical Practice. 8th edition. 2013. Chapter 140: Accidental Hypothermia. 1894-1895.*

#19

You are working as the base-camp physician on a climbing expedition. One of the climbers is being sent back down the mountain because of frostbite in her hands and feet. What would be INCORRECT?

A. Initiate prompt rewarming in the field en route with either hot water application or by friction massage.

B. Stabilize the core temperature, hydrate the patient and initiate rapid thawing at base camp/ED.

C. In the ED, thaw tissue rapidly and actively by immersion in circulating water that is 40-42°C.

D. Dry and elevate after full thaw, debride broken vesicles.

E. Consider tetanus prophylaxis and antibiotics against Streptococcus in severe cases.

#19

Answer: A

Field rewarming of frozen tissue is rarely practical. Greater damage to tissue can also occur if the rewarmed or partially rewarmed extremity or digit experiences refreezing in the field. Friction massage is contraindicated. Constricting or wet clothing should be removed and affected areas insulated and immobilized. Frostbite occurs when tissue temperature drops to less than 0°C and cellular damage results from ice-crystal formation, microvascular thrombosis, and stasis. All patients should be hospitalized for 24-48 hours to determine extent of injury, except in minor cases.

- *Rosen's Emergency Medicine - Concepts and Clinical Practice. 8th edition. 2013. Chapter 139: Frostbite. 1880.*

#20

Regarding submersion injuries, which of the following is FALSE?

A. The quantity of fluid aspirated rather than the composition (salt vs. fresh water) determines the subsequent pulmonary derangement.

B. The Heimlich maneuver should be used upon removal of the patient from submersion to help with removal of water from the lungs.

C. Antibiotics do not increase survival and should be administered only to the rare patient who was submerged in grossly contaminated water or shows signs of infection/sepsis.

D. Patient education in the ED can improve patient and family awareness to decrease the likelihood of recurrent events.

E. If indicated, CPR should proceed immediately upon removal of the patient from submersion.

#20

Answer B

While CPR should be initiated immediately in submersion victims even prior to complete extrication (in particular, rescue breathing), the use of the Heimlich maneuver is reserved for patients with a suspected airway obstruction by foreign body. The Heimlich maneuver is ineffective and dangerous in a victim at risk for aspiration. Its use may also delay ventilation support.

- *Rosen's Emergency Medicine - Concepts and Clinical Practice. 8th edition. 2013. Chapter 145: Drowning. 1943-1944.*

#21

Regarding electrical injuries and cardiac dysfunction, which of the following is FALSE?

A. Ventricular fibrillation is the most common arrhythmia causing death.

B. Acute electrical cardiac injury frequently results in sudden cardiac death due to asystole (usually with DC current or high voltage) or ventricular fibrillation (AC current).

C. Spontaneous return of sinus rhythm has been noted after asystole in these cases, but because respiratory paralysis lasts longer, the rhythm may degenerate to ventricular fibrillation.

D. Damage to the myocardium is uncommon but can occur as a result of heat injury or myocardial contusion resulting from the shock wave of a lightning strike.

E. Myocardial infarction is commonly seen.

#21

Answer: E

Damage to the myocardium is uncommon but can occur as a result of heat injury or myocardial contusion resulting from the shock wave of a lightning strike. Cardiac contusion is the most common pathologic cardiac finding, while myocardial infarction is rare. Other rare cardiac manifestations include coronary spasm and myocardial rupture due to coagulation necrosis, with arrhythmias occurring in 15% of cases. Cardiac injury usually results in sudden cardiac death due to asystole (usually with DC current or high voltage) or ventricular fibrillation (AC current) prior to hospital arrival.

Ventricular fibrillation is the most common fatal arrhythmia, occurring in up to 60% of patients in whom the current pathway goes from one hand to the other. Spontaneous return of sinus rhythm has been noted after asystole in these cases, but because respiratory paralysis lasts longer, the rhythm may degenerate to ventricular fibrillation. Atrial arrhythmias, first and second-degree heart block, and bundle branch blocks have been noted as well.

- *Rosen's Emergency Medicine - Concepts and Clinical Practice. 8th edition. 2013. Chapter 142: Electrical and Lightning Injuries. 1912-1913.*

#22

True statements about direct current (DC) electrical injuries include all of the following EXCEPT:

A. DC is used in items such as batteries, automobile electrical systems and high-voltage power lines.

B. Exposure to DC causes tetany that prolongs contact with the source, making it potentially more dangerous.

C. Ventricular fibrillation is more common with low voltage alternating current (AC) injuries.

D. Asystole is more commonly seen with DC high-voltage injuries.

E. Other initial ECG abnormalities reported with electrical injuries include sinus tachycardia, RBBB, 1st degree AV block, QT prolongation, PVCs, and atrial fibrillation.

#22

Answer: B

Most homes and offices use AC (alternating current) at a frequency of 60 cycles per second (Hz) in the United States and 50 Hz in Europe. Direct current only flows in one direction and causes a single muscle contraction that throws the victim away from the electrical source. With AC, there is prolonged tetany which increases contact with the source, making it potentially more dangerous.

Electrical injuries have three general clinical presentations:

1. Direct trauma from the electric current coursing through the body
2. Burns from conversion of electrical energy to thermal energy
3. Mechanical effects of the electric current, including violent muscle contractions and blunt trauma

- *Rosen's Emergency Medicine - Concepts and Clinical Practice. 8th edition. 2013. Chapter 142: Electrical and Lightning Injuries. 1907-1909.*

#23

Regarding lightning strikes, which of the following statements is FALSE?

A. Lightning strikes cause more deaths per year on average than any other storm conditions except for flooding.

B. Lightning behaves as an instantaneous massive, unidirectional current that is transmitted internally and then flashes over the body.

C. Cardiac arrest is the primary cause of mortality in lightning injury.

D. Lightning strikes commonly cause significant skin burns and soft tissue destruction.

E. Blunt injury is rarely a factor in morbidity from lightning strikes.

#23

Answer E

Lightning strikes frequently cause significant burns or soft tissue destruction. Cardiac arrest is the primary cause of mortality in lightning injury, and neurologic complications are the principal cause of morbidity. Keraunoparalysis is a transient (a few hours) neurologic paralysis that is pathognomonic for lightning injury. Keraunoparalysis is characterized by lower and occasionally upper extremities numbness, mottling and even pulselessness. The phenomenon is believed to be caused by transient vasospasm. Survival is good after a lightning strike if there is no cardiac or respiratory arrest.

In triaging lightning strike victims, the greatest priority should be for patients in cardiac or respiratory arrest. This is reversed from classic triage protocols. There is no intrinsic charge for people struck by lightning and they can be touched immediately. In addition to the cardiac injuries, blunt trauma is also common.

- *Rosen's Emergency Medicine - Concepts and Clinical Practice. 8th edition. 2013. Chapter 142: Electrical and Lightning Injuries. 1904-1911.*

#24

Field evaluation of lightning victims may involve triage of multiple victims. How does triage differ in the setting of lightning injury vs. other mass casualty incidents (MCI)?

A. They do not differ.

B. In lightning involved MCI, triage should initially focus on patients in cardiac arrest.

C. In lightning injuries, patients who are breathing spontaneously will get first priority.

D. None of the above

#24

Answer B

Cardiorespiratory arrest is the major cause of death in lightning injuries. Victims are likely to survive if they do not have cardiopulmonary arrest. Triage of lightning victims should concentrate on victims who appear to be in cardiac arrest. Those who are breathing spontaneously are likely to survive and can be triaged after the most critical patients who are in cardiac arrest.

- *Rosen's Emergency Medicine - Concepts and Clinical Practice. 8th edition. 2013. Chapter 142: Electrical and Lightning Injuries. 1913.*

#25

What are the factors that affect the magnitude of the blast overpressure and subsequent blast injury?

A. Medium in which the explosion takes place

B. Distance from the explosion

C. Whether or not one is in an open or closed space

D. All of the above

#25

Answer: D

The medium in which the explosion takes place affects blast injury. Water is non-compressible and blast waves in water propagate rapidly with a slow rate of dissipation. It has a greater potential for injury than explosions in air. The closer a patient is to an explosion, the greater the blast overpressure experienced. In a confined space, the maximum pressure can be reflected back from solid surfaces and increase its force.

- *Rosen's Emergency Medicine - Concepts and Clinical Practice. 8th edition. 2013. Chapter 193: Disaster Preparedness. 2477.*
- *Wolf SJ, et al. Blast injuries. Lancet. 2009 Aug 1;374(9687): 405-15. full text*

#26

You are seeing a patient who has severe hypothermia. What would you expect his urine output to be?

A. Decreased

B. Increased

C. Unchanged

#26

Answer: B

Simple exposure to cold induces a diuresis regardless of an individual's state of hydration. Hypothermia depresses renal blood flow, reducing it by 50% at 27 to 30 degrees Celsius. The kidneys then excrete a large amount of dilute urine, termed cold diuresis. Cold water immersion and ethanol ingestion can further increase urinary output.

- *Rosen's Emergency Medicine - Concepts and Clinical Practice. 8th edition. 2013. Chapter 140: Accidental Hypothermia. 1885.*

#27

You are seeing a patient who was scuba diving and now has symptoms of decompression sickness. What are the diving disorders that require recompression therapy?

(Choose three answers.)

A. Decompression sickness type I

B. Decompression sickness type II

C. Arterial gas embolism

D. Barodontalgia

#27

Answer: A, B, and C

Type I DCS (the bends) affects the musculoskeletal system, skin, and lymphatic vessels. Type II involves any other organ system and is more commonly reported and more serious (CNS, inner ear, and lungs). Recompression therapy is the only definitive treatment for DCS I and II, and arterial gas embolism (AGE). Hyperbaric therapy for AGE should be initiated as soon as possible for optimal results. Barodontalgia is dental pain that results from air that is trapped beneath a poorly filled dental cavity that expands on ascent. This condition is relatively benign and self-limited.

- *Rosen's Emergency Medicine - Concepts and Clinical Practice. 8th edition. 2013. Chapter 143: SCUBA Diving and Dysbarism. 1923-1925.*

#28

TRUE statements about snake envenomations include which of the following?

(Choose three answers.)

A. Dead snakes can envenomate careless handlers.

B. 100% of pit vipers have a pit midway between the eye and the nostril on both sides of the head.

C. The pit is a color-sensitive organ that enables snakes to see warm-blooded prey.

D. Typically, the pit vipers has a triangular head and an elliptical pupils, as well as fangs.

E. All of the above

#28

Answer: A, B, and D

In the identification of venomous snakes, two principles should be kept in mind. Only experts should handle live snakes, and even dead snakes can envenomate careless handlers. Pit vipers, have a characteristic pit midway between the eye and the nostril on both sides of the head. The pit is a heat-sensitive organ that enables it to locate warm-blooded prey. Pit vipers may be identified by other methods, but the presence of the pit is most reliable.

- *Rosen's Emergency Medicine - Concepts and Clinical Practice. 8th edition. 2013. Chapter 62: Venomous Animal Injuries. 794-799.*

#29

A 10 year old boy has been swimming and suffers a jellyfish sting. Which of the following may help relieve symptoms?

(Choose four answers.)

A. Pouring vinegar over the wound

B. Applying baking soda and alcohol on it

C. Immediately washing it with fresh water

D. Hot water immersion

E. Supportive pharmacologic therapy (analgesics, antihistamines, and steroid creams)

#29

Answer: A, B, D, and E

The best means of decreasing the pain of a jellyfish string is to remove the nematocyst prior to discharge. This is often more difficult than expected and requires small forceps and often magnification. There are many recommended regimens for treating stings however the effectiveness of each is species specific. Dilute acetic acid (vinegar) can deactivate the nematocysts. Baking soda and alcohol have also been reported as effective. In theory, fresh water should be avoided because it can activate the nematocysts. Hot water can relieve pain and supportive pharmacologic therapy in the form of opioids and NSAIDS will relieve pain. Although there are recommendations for various treatments based on region, there is little evidence based on good trials to suggest one method of treatment is superior to others. In general, however, avoid fresh water immersion.

- *Rosen's Emergency Medicine - Concepts and Clinical Practice. 8th edition. 2013. Chapter 62: Venomous Animal Injuries. 806-807.*

#30

Which of the following is TRUE about brown recluse spider envenomations?

(Choose three answers.)

A. There is an antivenin for Loxosceles available in the United States.

B. Dapsone has shown to be helpful in preventing local effects of the venom.

C. Systemic symptoms include fever, chills, rash, petechiae, nausea, vomiting, malaise and weakness.

D. The most common mimic of this necrotic spider bite is a Methicillin Resistant Staph Aureus (MRSA) skin infection.

#30

Answer: B, C, and D

An institute in Brazil produces an antivenin for Loxosceles bites, but it is not available in the United States. Hemolysis, thrombocytopenia, shock, jaundice, renal failure, hemorrhage, and pulmonary edema are a result of severe envenomation. Fatalities are more common in children. Dapsone, 50 to 200 mg/day may improved the pain and local swelling from the bite, but would not reverse the complications from a severe envenomation. Abscesses, especially those caused by MRSA can mimic the brown recluse wound.

- *Rosen's Emergency Medicine - Concepts and Clinical Practice. 8th edition. 2013. Chapter 62: Venomous Animal Injuries. 804.*

#31

A 29 year old pregnant woman presents to the ER after being bitten by one of her husband's pet black widow spiders (Latrodectus). Which of the following is FALSE?

A. Pregnant women, children and patients with cardiac disease should be admitted.

B. Antivenom should be administered to patients with severe envenomation, manifested as seizures, respiratory failure, uncontrolled hypertension, and in pregnant women.

C. Black widow is found throughout the Unites States, except for Alaska and in southern Canada.

D. The female spider is usually smaller than the male spider.

#31

Answer: D

The female spider is approximately twice as large as the male, and although both are venomous, only the female is a threat to humans. The venom depolarizes neuromuscular junctions by promoting the release of acetylcholine. All patients with symptoms of moderate envenomation, pregnant women, children, and those with cardiac disease should be admitted. Acute hypertensive problems should be treated with nitroprusside if diastolic pressure rises above 120 mmHg. Pregnant women may experience premature labor. Peritonitis is also a possible manifestation in severe bites. Symptom control from local pain and muscle cramping are the most common focus of supportive care.

- *Rosen's Emergency Medicine - Concepts and Clinical Practice. 8th edition. 2013. Chapter 62: Venomous Animal Injuries. 803-804.*

#32

TRUE statements about immersion syndrome include which of the following?

A. Wetting the face before entering the water may prevent it.

B. The risk of immersion syndrome is proportional to the difference between body and water temperature.

C. Both of the above

D. Neither of the above

#32

Answer: C

Immersion syndrome specifically refers to syncope caused by asystole due to vagal stimulation or ventricular fibrillation secondary to QT prolongation. The cold water may also induce a catecholamine surge, and the loss of consciousness leads to drowning. Generally the syndrome is thought to occur when there is a 5 degree difference between body temperature and water.

- *Rosen's Emergency Medicine - Concepts and Clinical Practice. 8th edition. 2013. Chapter 145: Drowning. 1941-1942.*

#33

True or False: The diving reflex may play a protective role in infant and child submersions.

A. True

B. False

#33

Answer: A

True. The diving reflex causes shunting of blood centrally to the heart and brain and causes apnea and bradycardia. This event may prolong the ability to survive a prolonged submersion.

- *Rosen's Emergency Medicine - Concepts and Clinical Practice. 8th edition. 2013. Chapter 145: Drowning. 1942.*

#34

What should be the disposition of a 6 year old child who had a submersion injury but is asymptomatic on presentation to the ED, has a oxygen saturation of 98%, and has a normal chest X-ray and blood gas?

A. Discharge after the chest X-ray results

B. Discharge after 12 hours of observation

C. Admit

D. Discharge after 6 hours of observation

#34

Answer: D

It is always safe to allow for 6 hours of observation in patients who have had a submersion event. Symptomatic patients should be admitted. Admission should be considered if there was a history of unconsciousness, hypoxia, dysrhythmia or chest X-ray abnormality. If a patient has an uneventful ED course and has good followup and home support, then discharge after observation is appropriate. All patients going home should receive instructions regarding delayed pulmonary complications.

- *Rosen's Emergency Medicine - Concepts and Clinical Practice. 8th edition. 2013. Chapter 145: Drowning. 1944.*

#35

In the hypothermic coagulopathic patient above, the treatment of choice is:

A. Administration of clotting factors

B. Rewarming

C. Both of the above

D. Neither of the above

#35

Answer: B

The most effective treatment is rewarming, not the administration of clotting factors.

- *Rosen's Emergency Medicine - Concepts and Clinical Practice. 8th edition. 2013. Chapter 140: Accidental Hypothermia. 1888-1890.*

#36

True or False: If the patient's temperature is not above 40.5°C (105°F) in the ED, then the patient can not have heat stroke.

A. True

B. False

#36

Answer: B

The usual manifestations of heatstroke include hyperpyrexia above 40.5°C, altered mental status and hot flushed skin with or without sweating. Patients can be cooled below the initial temperature during transport and may present with a temperature less than 40.5°C (105°F).

- *Rosen's Emergency Medicine - Concepts and Clinical Practice. 8th edition. 2013. Chapter 141: Heat Illness. 1903.*

#37

If the electrical currents involve the same voltage, which of the following is more dangerous?

A. Alternating Current (AC)

B. Direct Current (DC)

C. They are the same.

#37

Answer: A

One of the factors affecting the nature and severity of electrical injury is the type of circuit involved, either direct current or alternating current. High-voltage DC often causes a single muscle spasm. This spasm can even throw the patient from the source causing other associated injuries. However, when a victim is thrown, it theoretically creates a shorter duration of current exposure. The DC source can also cause cardiac arrhythmias, depending on the phase of the cardiac cycle affected. In contrast, AC exposure of the same voltage can be three times more dangerous than DC, due to the alternating current causing prolonged and continuous muscle contraction and tetany. The tetany results in longer electrical exposure.

- *Rosen's Emergency Medicine - Concepts and Clinical Practice. 8th edition. 2013. Chapter 142: Electrical and Lightning Injuries. 1906.*

#38

Factors determining the degree of harm in an electrical injury include which of the following?

A. Duration of exposure or contact

B. Resistance of tissues

C. Voltage

D. Amperage

E. Pathway of current

F. All of the above

#38

Answer: F

The greater the resistance, the greater the transformation of electrical energy into thermal energy. Current, expressed in amperes, is a measure of the amount of energy that flows through an object. The heat generated is proportional to the amperage squared. The longer the duration of contact with high-voltage current, the greater the heat causing tissue destruction. Voltage is a measure of the difference in electrical potential between two points and is determined by the electrical source.

Electrical injuries can be categorized as low (<1000 volts) or high voltage (>1000 volts). The systems injured is determined by the pathway through the body. Current passing through the heart can cause arrhythmias and infarction, and current through the brain can cause seizures, and respiratory arrest.

- *Rosen's Emergency Medicine - Concepts and Clinical Practice. 8th edition. 2013. Chapter 142: Electrical and Lightning Injuries. 1906-1914.*

#39

A 5 year old male accidentally had his head under the water for 10 seconds and comes up WITHOUT any respiratory impairment. This should be classified as:

A. Drowning

B. Near drowning

C. Delayed onset respiratory distress

D. Nonfatal drowning

E. Water rescue

#39

Answer: E

The WHO defines "drowning as the process of experiencing respiratory impairment from submersion/immersion in liquid. If a person is rescued at any time, the process of drowning is interrupted, and it is termed a nonfatal drowning. If the person dies at any time as a result of drowning, this is termed a fatal drowning. Any submersion or immersion incident without evidence of respiratory impairment should be considered a water rescue and not a drowning. Terms such as "near drowning," "dry or wet drowning," "secondary drowning," etc. should be avoided.

- *Szpilman D, et al. Drowning. N Engl J Med. 2012 May 31; 366(22): 2102-10. full text*

#40

You are taking care of a patient who has drowned. The patient appears to be in cardiac arrest. Which of the following steps should be taken?

A. CPR following the traditional airway-breathing-circulation sequence

B. CPR following the newly recommended circulation-airway-breathing sequence

C. CPR with chest compression only

D. Expel water from the airway by means of abdominal thrusts or placing the person head down

#40

Answer: A

Cardiac arrest from downing is due primarily to lack of oxygen. CPR should follow the traditional ABC sequence, starting with five initial rescue breaths, followed by 30 chest compressions, and continuing with two rescue breaths and 30 compressions until signs of life appear, the rescuer becomes exhausted, or ALS becomes available. The most frequent complication during a resuscitation attempt is the regurgitation of stomach contents. Active efforts to expel water from the airway should be avoided because they delay the initiation of ventilation and increase the risk of vomiting and mortality. CPR with chest compression ONLY is NOT advised in persons who have drowned.

- *Szpilman D, et al. Drowning. N Engl J Med. 2012 May 31; 366(22): 2102-10. full text*

#41

Which of the following are important predictors of outcome in resuscitation of a person who has drowned?

A. Age

B. Whether it was fresh or salt water

C. Duration of submersion

D. None of the above

#41

Answer: C

Important facts and predictors of outcome in resuscitation of a person who has drowned include the following:

1. Availability of early basic and advance life support
2. Reduction of brain temperature
3. Duration of submersion
4. Signs of brainstem injury

There is an estimated 10% risk of death or severe neurologic impairment if the duration of submersion is 0-5 minutes. The risk increases to near 100% as submersion times approach 25 minutes. Each reduction in brain temperature by 10 degrees decreases ATP consumption by 50% and doubles the duration of time that the brain can survive. Therefore, colder water may offer a degree of neuroprotection.

- *Szpilman D, et al. Drowning. N Engl J Med. 2012 May 31; 366(22): 2102-10. full text*

#42

Which of the following patients after drowning can be discharged home?

A. Patient with normal oxygenation, lung exam, but with a cough

B. Patient with rales

C. Patient with grade 2-4 injury

D. None of the above

#42

Answer: A

Patients who have good arterial oxygenation without need for supplemental oxygen and who have no other associated injuries can be safely discharged. Hospitalization is recommended for all patients with a presentation of grade 2 (patient in answer B) to 6. For most patients with grade 2 presentation, noninvasive oxygen administration results in normalization oxygenation and can be discharged after 6-8 hrs of observation. Patients with grade 3-6 usually need intubation, mechanical ventilation, and hospitalization in an ICU.

Grade 1—normal pulmonary auscultation with coughing

Grade 2—abnormal pulmonary auscultation with rales in some pulmonary fields

Grade 3—acute pulmonary edema without arterial hypotension

Grade 4—acute pulmonary edema with arterial hypotension

Grade 5—isolated respiratory arrest

Grade 6—cardiopulmonary arrest.

- *Szpilman D, et al. Drowning. N Engl J Med. 2012 May 31; 366(22): 2102-10. full text*

#43

With respect to nonfatal drowning incidents, the clinical picture is determined predominantly by which of the following?

A. Whether it was salt or fresh water

B. The amount of water that has been aspirated and its effects

C. Both of the above

D. Neither of the above

#43

Answer: B

If the person is rescued alive, the clinical picture is determined predominantly by the amount of water that has been aspirated and its effects. Water in the alveoli causes surfactant dysfunction and washout. Aspiration of salt water and aspiration of freshwater cause similar degrees of injury, although with difference in osmotic gradients. The combined effects of fluids in the lungs, loss of surfactant, and increased permeability of the alveolar-capillary membrane result in decreased lung compliance, increased regions of low ventilation to perfusion in the lungs, atelectasis, and bronchospasm.

- *Szpilman D, et al. Drowning. N Engl J Med. 2012 May 31; 366(22): 2102-10. full text*

#44

Regarding nonfatal drowning incidents, which of the following is TRUE?

A. Injuries to the cervical spine occur in approximately 10%, so immobilization of the spine is indicated in all patients.

B. The rate of cerebral oxygen consumption is reduced by approximately 5% for each 1 degree Celsius reduction in temperature within the range of 37 to 20 degrees.

C. When rescuing a person from the water, rescuers should try to maintain the person in a horizontal position while keeping the airway open.

#44

Answer: B

If CPR is required, the risk of neurologic damage is similar to that in other instances of cardiac arrest. However, hypothermia associated with drowning can provide a protective mechanism that allows persons to survive prolonged submersion episodes. Injuries to the C-spine occur in less than 0.5% of persons who are drowning, and immobilization of the spine in the water is indicated only in cases in which head or neck injury is strongly suspected. When rescuing a person from the water, the rescuer should try to maintain the person in a vertical position while keeping the airway open, which helps to prevent vomiting and further aspiration of water and stomach contents.

- *Szpilman D, et al. Drowning. N Engl J Med. 2012 May 31; 366(22): 2102-10. full text*

- *Rosen's Emergency Medicine - Concepts and Clinical Practice. 8th edition. 2013. Chapter 145: Drowning. 1941-1942.*

#45

Regarding nonfatal drowning, which of the following is TRUE?

(Choose two answers.)

A. If the patient is in cardiac arrest, CPR should follow the circulation -> airway -> breathing sequence.

B. CPR should be continued until the patient has been rewarmed and asystole has persisted for > 20 minutes.

C. Metabolic alkalosis occurs in the majority of patients.

D. In most persons who have been rescued from drowning, the circulation becomes adequate after oxygenation, rapid crystalloid infusion, and restoration of normal body temperature.

E. Presenting rhythm in cases of cardiac arrest after drowning is usually ventricular fibrillation.

#45

Answer: B and D

Cardiac arrest from drowning is due primarily to lack of oxygen. For this reason, it is important that CPR follow the traditional airway-breathing-circulation (ABC) sequence, rather than the circulation-airway-breathing (CAB) sequence, starting with five initial rescue breaths, followed by 30 chest compressions and continuing with two rescue breaths and 30 compressions until signs of life reappear. CPR with chest compression only is not advised in persons who have drowned. Metabolic acidosis occurs in the majority of patients and is usually corrected by the patient's spontaneous effort to increase minute ventilation or by setting a higher minute ventilation or a higher peak inspiratory pressure. The presenting rhythm in cases of cardiac arrest is usually asystole or pulseless electrical activity.

- *Szpilman D, et al. Drowning. N Engl J Med. 2012 May 31; 366(22): 2102-10. full text*
- *Rosen's Emergency Medicine - Concepts and Clinical Practice. 8th edition. 2013. Chapter 145: Drowning. 1943-1944.*

#46

Primary blast injuries happen most frequently in what organ systems?

(Choose three answers.)

A. Endocrine

B. Hematologic

C. Pulmonary

D. Gastrointestinal

E. Auditory

#46

Answer: C, D, and E

Primary blast injuries take place when the blast overpressure reaches the person and transmitted forces exert their effect on the body. These occur with greatest frequency at air-tissue interfaces. Thus, organ systems with high air content, such as the pulmonary, GI, and auditory systems are the most susceptible. The auditory system is the system most commonly affected by blast overpressure (tympanic membrane ruptures).

- *LLSA 2013: Wolf SJ, et al. Blast injuries. Lancet; 2009 Aug 1; 374(9687): 405-15. full text*

#47

Match the appropriate type of blast injury (primary, secondary, tertiary, or quaternary) with the patient.

Blast Injury:

1. Primary
2. Secondary
3. Tertiary
4. Quaternary

Patient:

A. Patient who has a nail and scrap metal puncture wound

B. Patient who was thrown from a pressure wave and sustained a head injury

C. Crush injury

D. Burns, toxic substance exposure

E. Psychological trauma

#47

Answer:

A = 2 (Secondary)

B = 3 (Tertiary)

C = 3 (Tertiary)

D = 4 (Quaternary)

E = 4 (Quaternary)

Primary blast injuries are caused by direct tissue and organ damage from blast force transmission. Secondary blast injuries are created by debris that is physically injures the patient. Tertiary blast injuries are caused when a person is displaced by the blast force and sustains blunt trauma. Finally, quaternary blast injuries are caused directly by the explosion but are not classified as primary, secondary, or tertiary injuries. These include burns, toxic substance exposures, and psychological trauma.

- *LLSA 2013: Wolf SJ, et al. Blast injuries. Lancet; 2009 Aug 1; 374(9687): 405-15. full text*

GASTROENTERO-LOGY

#1

Which of the following statements about appendicitis is TRUE?

A. There is no value of total WBC count that has sufficient sensitivity and specificity to be of clinical value in the diagnosis of appendicitis.

B. There is no value of a specific temperature that has sufficient sensitivity and specificity to be of clinical value in the diagnosis of appendicitis.

C. Clinicians should be wary of reliance on either elevated temperature or total WBC count as an indicator of the presence of appendicitis.

D. The total white blood cell (WBC) count and temperature are often expected to be elevated in patients with appendicitis.

E. All of the above statements are true.

#1

Answer: E

In 2004, Cardall T, et al. assessed the discriminatory value of the total WBC count and temperature in patients presenting to the emergency department (ED) with signs and symptoms suggestive of appendicitis.

In this study group of patients:

A total WBC count >10,000 cells/mm3 had a:

- Sensitivity of 76% (95% confidence interval [95% CI] = 65% to 84%)
- Specificity of 52% (95% CI = 45% to 60%)
- Positive predictive value (PPV) of 42% (95% CI = 35% to 51%)
- Negative predictive value (NPV) of 82% (95% CI = 74% to 89%)
- Positive likelihood ratio (LR) of 1.59 (95% CI = 1.31 to 1.93)
- Negative LR of 0.46 (95% CI = 0.31 to 0.67)

A temperature > 99.0 °F had a:

- Sensitivity of 47% (95% CI 36%-57%)
- Specificity of 64% (95% CI 57%-71%)
- PPV of 37% (95% CI 29%-46%)
- NPV of 72% (95% CI 65%-79%)
- Positive LR was 1.3 (95% CI 0.97-1.72)
- Negative LR was 0.82 (95% CI 0.65-1.01)

The areas under the curve for the receiver-operating characteristic (ROC) curve were 0.72 (95% CI = 0.65 to 0.79) and 0.59 (95% CI = 0.52 to 0.66) for an elevated total WBC count and an elevated temperature, respectively.

The authors conclude that an elevated total WBC count >10,000, while statistically associated with the presence of appendicitis, had very poor sensitivity and specificity and almost no clinical utility.

For area under ROC curve, an area of 1 represents a perfect test and an area of 0.5 represents a useless test. A guide for interpreting values between 0.5-1 are:

0.90-1 = excellent

0.80-0.90 = good

0.70-0.80 = fair

0.60-0.70 = poor

0.50-0.60 = not useful

- *Cardall T, et al. Clinical value of the total white blood cell count and temperature in the evaluation of patients with suspected appendicitis. Acad Emerg Med. 2004 Oct; 11(10): 1021-7. full text*

#2

Regarding diverticular disease, which of the following is FALSE?

A. Patients with acute diverticulitis classically present with severe, constant left lower quadrant pain, localized tenderness, fever, and leukocytosis.

B. Most patients with diverticulosis are asymptomatic.

C. Patients with diverticulosis may present with painless, massive rectal bleeding.

D. Diverticulosis is more likely to require surgery in older patients than in younger patients.

E. Indications for admission include disease complicated by abscess, fistula formation, obstruction, perforation, or significant comorbidities or immunodeficiency.

#2

Answer: D

Although less frequently encountered in patients younger than 40 years of age, diverticulosis is relatively more likely to be complicated and require surgery in younger patients than in older patients. Patients with diverticulitis complicated by abscess or fistula formation, obstruction, or perforation should be admitted, as well as patients suspected of having severe acute diverticulitis and those with gross lower GI bleeding. Outpatient management should be limited to immunocompetent patients with mild uncomplicated diverticulitis.

- *Rosen's Emergency Medicine - Concepts and Clinical Practice. 8th edition. 2013. Chapter 95: Disorders of the Large Intestine. 1262-1265.*

- *Weizman AV, Nguyen GC. Diverticular disease: epidemiology and management. Can J Gastroenterol. 2011 Jul; 25(7): 385-9. full text*

#3

The most common location of the appendix is:

A. Retrocecal

B. Pelvic

C. Subcecal

D. Preileal

E. Paracolic

F. Postileal

#3

Answer: A

In a classic study of 10,000 post-mortem cases of appendicitis, retrocecal was the most common location (65%). The length ranged from 2-20 cm with an average length of 9 cm. The innervation is from the autonomic nervous system. No somatic pain fibers are found in the appendix itself. The pain is poorly localized initially but when the adjacent parietal peritoneum becomes inflamed, the somatic pain fibers are activated and the pain becomes more localized.

- *Wakeley CPG. The position of the vermiform appendix as ascertained by an analysis of 10000 cases. J Anat. 1933;67:277–83. full text*

#4

Several scoring systems exist with the goal of identifying patients in whom the diagnosis of appendicitis is likely. The most widely known scoring system is the Alvarado/MANTRELS score. Which of the following is not a component of this scoring system?

A. Nausea/Vomiting

B. Right lower quadrant tenderness

C. Rebound pain

D. Leukocytosis

E. All of the above are components of the Alvarado score.

#4

Answer: E

The Alvarado score assigns values to:

Symptoms:

1. Migration or pain to the right lower quadrant (RLQ)
2. Anorexia
3. Nausea/vomiting
4. Right lower quadrant tenderness
5. Rebound pain
6. Elevation of temperature > 37.3°C)

Laboratory findings:

1. Leukocytosis > 10,000 /mm3
2. Left shift > 75% neutrophils

The total score is 10. Patients with Alvarado scores of ≥ 7 have a likelihood of acute appendicitis of 77-93% and < 3 have a likelihood of 4-6%.

- *Alvarado, A. A Practical Score for the Early Diagnosis of Acute Appendicitis. Ann Emerg Med. 1986; 15(5): 557–64. full text*

#5

Regarding acute pancreatitis, the following statements are true EXCEPT:

A. The majority of all cases are caused by either gallstones or alcoholism. Other etiologies include hyperlipidemia, drugs, scorpion bites, viral/bacterial and post operative/post procedural.

B. Multi-organ complications/systemic injury arise from direct release of pancreatic enzymes into the bloodstream and initiation of the systemic inflammatory response.

C. Serum lipase, compared to amylase, has equivalent sensitivity with higher specificity. It also has an earlier rise and peak in serum levels.

D. The degree of elevation of amylase or lipase is a marker of disease severity.

E. Elevations in aspartate transaminase and LDH portend to a worse prognosis.

#5

Answer: D

While the etiology of pancreatitis favors alcoholism and gallstones, up to 10% of cases are idiopathic in nature. Complications include shock from volume loss, hemorrhage or fluid sequestration. The degree of elevation of serum (amylase/lipase) markers is not an indicator of disease severity. In fact, alcoholics frequently have lower amylase levels but may develop more severe disease than non alcoholic patients. Ranson's criteria is a two-step list of laboratory values, determined at admission and then at 48 hours after admission to predict in-hospital mortality.

- *Rosen's Emergency Medicine - Concepts and Clinical Practice. 8th edition. 2013. Chapter 91: Disorders of the Pancreas. 1205-1210.*

#6

A 40 year old female presents with fever, chills, nausea, vomiting and abdominal pain in the right upper quadrant. Vital signs are: 101°F, BP 98/65, HR 102. In differentiating acute cholecystitis from cholangitis, which of the following would be helpful?

A. WBC with a left shift

B. Fever

C. Jaundice

D. Elevated alkaline phosphatase

E. Elevated aminotransferases and bilirubin

#6

Answer: C

Cholangitis can be caused by common bile duct obstruction from a gallstone, malignancy or anatomic stricture. The obstruction then leads to increased intraluminal pressure and bacterial infection. Most obstructions in cholangitis are incomplete and involve E. coli, Klebsiella, Enterococcus, and Bacteroides.

Charcot's triad of right upper quadrant pain, fever and jaundice may present along with fever, chills, nausea, vomiting. Sepsis is a common complication (Charcot's triad plus sepsis and altered sensorium equals Reynold's pentad). The presence of jaundice is the clinical sign most helpful in differentiating cholangitis from cholecystitis.

- *Rosen's Emergency Medicine - Concepts and Clinical Practice. 8th edition. 2013. Chapter 90: Disorders of the Liver and Biliary Tract. 1203-1204.*

#7

Regarding mesenteric ischemia, all of the following are true, EXCEPT:

A. The most common cause is arterial embolus, accounting for approximately 50% of cases.

B. Abdominal CT scan with IV contrast is the gold standard for diagnosis.

C. Elevated serum lactate level is a highly sensitive test for mesenteric ischemia.

D. Supine and upright plain films are appropriate to initially evaluate for obstruction or free air.

E. Arterial thrombosis and non-occlusive vascular disease are causes of mesenteric ischemia.

#7

Answer: B

Acute mesenteric ischemia is caused by arterial embolus (50%), arterial thrombosis (15%), venous occlusion (15%) and non-occlusive vascular disease (20%). Early diagnosis and aggressive intervention is crucial given mortality rates range from 70-90% when infarction occurs. CT scanning is capable of demonstrating bowel edema, abnormal gas patterns, intramural gas and occasionally evidence of mesenteric venous thrombosis. However, angiography still remains the gold standard to diagnose mesenteric ischemia.

- *Rosen's Emergency Medicine - Concepts and Clinical Practice. 8th edition. 2013. Chapter 92: Disorders of the Small Intestine. 1221-1224.*

#8

A CT scan obtained in a patient with abdominal pain demonstrates diverticulitis without perforation, abscess or obstruction. In consultation with your surgical colleagues, you have determined that the patient does not need hospitalization. His outpatient management should include all of the following EXCEPT:

A. Oral antibiotics covering E. coli and B. fragilis

B. A diet that is high in fiber

C. A clear liquid diet

D. Precautions to return if there is fever, vomiting, or increased abdominal pain

E. A follow-up appointment for a recheck in 24-48 hours

#8

Answer: B

Outpatients should be instructed to consume clear liquids only with the diet advanced after 3 days if there is improvement. Patients requiring hospitalization can be treated with clear liquids or NPO with intravenous hydration. The choice of antibiotics should be based upon the usual bacteria, which are generally gram negative rods and anaerobes (particularly E. coli and B. fragilis). Ciprofloxacin and metronidazole are the usual combination. Outpatients should be advised to return for increasing pain, fever, or the inability to tolerate fluids, all of which may be an indication for hospitalization.

The natural history of the diverticulitis has shown that one third of patients will remain asymptomatic, one third will have episodic abdominal cramps without frank diverticulitis, and one-third will proceed to a second attack of diverticulitis.

- *Friend K, Mills AM. Is outpatient oral antibiotic therapy safe and effective for the treatment of acute uncomplicated diverticulitis? Ann Emerg Med. 2011 Jun;57(6): 600-2.*

#9

You are seeing a patient with ascites secondary to cirrhosis. You have performed a therapeutic paracentesis and are ready to discharge him from the ED. Which of the following are NOT thought to be helpful in preventing reaccumulation of ascites and other complications of liver disease?

A. NSAID administration

B. Spironolactone/diuretics

C. Low sodium diet (2000mg/day)

D. Avoidance of hypokalemia

E. Abstinence from alcohol

#9

Answer: A

Dietary sodium restriction is important in the management of cirrhotic ascites. Patients should also avoid non-steroidal anti-inflammatory drugs (NSAIDs), which can impair renal function by increasing vasoconstriction. In patients who require diuretic therapy, combined therapy with spironolactone and lasix is beneficial. Hypokalemia can increase renal ammonia production and possibly induce hepatic encephalopathy. Obviously, further alcohol consumption worsens hepatic function.

- *Rosen's Emergency Medicine - Concepts and Clinical Practice. 8th edition. 2013. Chapter 90: Disorders of the Liver and Biliary Tract. 1193-1194.*

#10

You are seeing a patient with end-stage liver disease secondary to alcoholic cirrhosis, and he asks you for pain medications after he sprained his ankle. Which of the following would be the best treatment option?

A. NSAIDS

B. Acetaminophen

C. Codeine

D. Toradol

E. Aspirin

#10

Answer: B

Acetaminophen is actually an effective and safe analgesic for patients with chronic liver disease when used at low doses. For patients with ongoing alcohol ingestion and cirrhosis, acetaminophen may be used at a maximum of 2-3 grams per day, which is less than the normal recommended daily dosage. NSAIDs are associated with an increased risk of variceal hemorrhage, impaired renal function, and the development of diuretic resistant ascites. Thus, NSAIDs, including aspirin, should be avoided in cirrhotics. Opioids should also be used cautiously in cirrhotics and usually at lower doses, especially codeine, which can have variable metabolism.

- *Chandok, N, Watt K. Pain Management in the Cirrhotic Patient: The Clinical Challenge. Mayo Clin Proc. May 2010; 85(5): 451–458. full text*

#11

You suspect that a patient of yours has acute viral hepatitis and you would like to send some tests to determine which type of hepatitis. All of the following serologies would be indicated EXCEPT:

A. Hepatitis A IgG antibody

B. Hepatitis A IgM antibody

C. Hepatitis B surface antigen

D. Hepatitis B core IgM antibody

E. Hepatitis C viral RNA

#11

Answer: A

IgG antibodies indicate immunization or a past infection, thus Hepatitis A IgG antibody would not be useful. The other serologies would be helpful, if positive. Clinically, acute hepatitis C is often silent until sequelae of cirrhosis develop. In a patient with risk factors, HCV testing should be performed. The viral RNA Hepatitis C antibody may be undetectable early in an acute infection.

- *Rosen's Emergency Medicine - Concepts and Clinical Practice. 8th edition. 2013. Chapter 90: Disorders of the Liver and Biliary Tract. 1187-1188.*

#12

The most common oral manifestation of Crohn's disease is:

A. Aphthous ulcers

B. Granulomatous nodules

C. Cheilitis

D. Granulomatous sialadenitis

E. Herpes gingivostomatitis

#12

Answer: A

Aphthous ulcers are the most common oral manifestation of Crohn's disease. Other less common oral lesions are granulomatous cheilitis and sialadenitis. The greatest complication is decreased oral intake, dehydration and poor nutrition due to the pain from the lesions. Treatment is generally supportive with topical carafate; oral lesions abate with treatment of the intestinal disease.

- *Jurge S, et al. Recurrent aphthous stomatitis. Oral Dis. 2006 Jan; 12(1): 1-21.*
- *Nayar M, Rhodes JM Management of inflammatory bowel disease. Postgrad Med J. 2004 Apr;80(942):206-13. full text*

#13

TRUE statements about Crohn's disease involving the perianal area include which of the following:

A. One-third of patients with Crohn's disease will manifest perianal lesions, such as abscesses and fistulae.

B. In a draining fistulae or small abscesses not amenable to surgical drainage, 10 mg/kg of Flagyl per day may be effective.

C. It is important to establish the extent of the fistula tract either through advanced imaging, to exclude abscesses, and to evaluate for the presence of inflammation of the rectal mucosa.

D. All of the above

#13

Answer: D

All of the statements about perianal manifestations of Crohn's disease are true. The paper by Safar and Sands linked below provides a great review of perianal disease in Crohn's.

- *Rosen's Emergency Medicine - Concepts and Clinical Practice. 8th edition. 2013. Chapter 95: Disorders of the Large Intestine. 1270-1272.*

- *Safar B, Sands D. Perianal Crohn's disease. Clin Colon Rectal Surg. 2007 Nov; 20(4): 282-93. full text*

#14

A patient with known ulcerative colitis presents with tenesmus due to ulcerative proctitis. What would be the best management strategy?

A. Sitz baths

B. Anusol cream

C. Lidocaine suppositories

D. Surgery

E. 5-ASA suppositories

#14

Answer: E

Ulcerative proctitis refers to disease limited to the rectum. The mainstay of therapy for ulcerative proctitis is the topical administration of 5-aminosalicylate (5-ASA) suppositories or steroid foams.

.Cottone M, et al. Is 5-ASA still the treatment of choice for ulcerative colitis? Curr Drug Targets. 2011 Sep;12(10): 1396-405.

#15

In the patient who presents with acute abdominal pain, opiate administration:

A. Does not alter the physical examination findings

B. Increases morbidity

C. Increases mortality

D. May alter the physical exam findings but does not significantly change the rate of management errors.

E. Is contraindicated in all cases.

#15

Answer: D

Traditionally patient with acute abdominal pain were not given opioids so the abdominal exam would not be altered and interfere with a potential surgical diagnosis. In a systematic review of studies both in adults (9 trials) and in children (3 trials), there were trends toward increased risks of altered findings on the abdominal examination due to opiate administration, with risk ratios for changes in the examination of 1.51 (95% CI, 0.85 to 2.69) and 2.11 (95% CI, 0.60 to 7.35), respectively.

Opiate administration had no significant association with management errors (+0.3% absolute increase; 95% CI, -4.1% to +4.7%). The 3 pediatric trials showed a nonsignificant absolute decrease in management errors (-0.8%; 95% CI, -8.6% to +6.9%). Across adult and pediatric trials with adequate analgesia, opiate administration was associated with a nonsignificant absolute decrease in the risk of management errors (-0.2%; 95% CI, -4.0% to +3.6%). Thus, opiate administration may alter the physical examination finding but does not cause management errors. No patient suffered morbidity or mortality attributable to opiate administration.

- *Ranji SR, et al. Do opiates affect the abdominal examination? JAMA. 2006 Oct 11;296(14): 1764-74. full text*

#16

The most common surgical procedure performed for morbid obesity to promote weight loss in the United States today is:

A. Roux-en-Y Gastric bypass

B. Biliopancreatic diversion

C. Vertical banded gastroplasty

D. Laparoscopic adjustable gastric banding

E. Gastrectomy

#16

Answer: A

The Roux-en-Y gastric bypass is the most commonly performed operation for morbid obesity. It restricts the amount of food able to be consumed in a single sitting and also creates malabsorption which promotes further weight loss. Roux-en-Y has been shown to produce and maintain excess weight loss of 60% to 80% at 5 years.

- *Edwards ED, et al. Presentation and management of common post-weight loss surgery problems in the emergency department. Ann Emerg Med. 2006 Feb; 47(2): 160-6. full text*

#17

Complications after Roux-en-Y gastric bypass include which of the following:

A. Obstruction due to strictures

B. Small bowel herniation

C. Anastomotic leak

D. Acute gastric dilation

E. All of the above

#17

Answer: E

Early complications include anastomotic leak, intra-abdominal bleeding, and deep venous thrombosis or pulmonary embolism. Any patient who presents in the first weeks after a Roux-en-Y with tachycardia and fever should be suspected of an anastomotic leak or intraabdominal abscess.

Patients can also develop gastric dilation due to Roux limb obstruction. Presenting complaints will be similar to a small bowel obstruction. Bleeding along the surgical sites and staple line at the gastrojejunostomy (most common), the jejunojejunostomy and even along the transected edge of the gastric remnant are possible.

Late complications of Roux-en-Y can be divided into anatomic and systemic complications. Patients develop bowel obstructions from adhesions, anastomotic strictures or internal hernias. The internal hernia occurs when a portion of small bowel herniates through the mesenteric defect between the transverse colon and the Roux limb. S

Systemic complications include nutritional deficiencies in iron, vitamin B12, vitamin D, and calcium. Patients also develop secondary hyperparathyroidism and show increased bone turnover and decreased bone density.

- *Edwards ED, et al. Presentation and management of common post-weight loss surgery problems in the emergency department. Ann Emerg Med. 2006 Feb; 47(2): 160-6. full text*

#18

A 35 year old obese female patient who underwent a laparoscopic adjustable gastric banding (LAP-BAND) procedure 3 months prior to presentation for weight loss, presents with intractable nausea and vomiting streaked with blood, consistent with an obstruction. She states that the "balloon was inflated more yesterday." What is the next best step in management?

A. Call surgery, requesting to assist in deflating the lap band balloon as quickly as possible.

B. Place a foley catheter.

C. Place a rectal tube for decompression.

D. Give her some water oral challenge challenge.

E. Leave her chart for the next emergency physician coming on-shift.

#18

Answer: A

Laparoscopic adjustable gastric banding is a common technique used in the surgical treatment of morbid obesity. There are two main devices approved by the US Food and Drug Administration, on the market, the LAP-BAND (FDA approval 2001) and the REALIZE Band (FDA approval 2007). The devices consist of an adjustable silastic band that is positioned around the upper portion of the stomach.

Mechanical problems with the bands may occur, including breakage, infection, and even erosion of the band into the gastrointestinal tract. Migration of the band can cause gastric dilatation with nausea and vomiting. Migration is also referred to as "slippage" and involves movement of the band to a different portion of the stomach.

Depending on the acuity of the patient, emergent deflation of the band can be performed in the emergency department, in consultation with the surgeon. Early deflation can prevent the band from progressing from erosion to perforation. The band can be deflated by infiltrating the overlying skin with lidocaine, stabilizing the port between 2 fingers, and then accessing the port with a large-bore needle.

- *Edwards ED, et al. Presentation and management of common post-weight loss surgery problems in the emergency department. Ann Emerg Med. 2006 Feb; 47(2): 160-6. full text*

#19

A 55 year old patient with a long history of alcoholic cirrhosis and recurrent ascites presents with increased abdominal girth. On examination, he has tense ascites and diffuse tenderness to palpation. You are concerned about spontaneous bacterial peritonitis, and you are preparing to perform a paracentesis. The nurse calls you to notify you that his INR is 2.2, platelet count is 45/µL, and hemoglobin is 11g/dL. You should:

A. Delay the paracentesis since he is coagulopathic.

B. Perform the paracentesis only after administering platelets.

C. Perform the paracentesis only after administering fresh frozen plasma.

D. Perform the paracentesis under ultrasound guidance.

E. Administer vitamin K and DDAVP.

#19

Answer: D

Many patients that require paracentesis have coagulopathy or thrombocytopenia as a result of underlying liver disease. However, clinically significant bleeding complications is rare (a recent retrospective study of more than 4500 paracenteses reported severe hemorrhage in < 0.2% of procedures) and reversal with Fresh Frozen Plasma prior to performing the procedure is not recommended. Patients should be observed after the procedure to assess for any bleeding complications.

- *Thomsen TW. Paracentesis. N Engl J Med. 2006 Nov 9; 355(19):e21.*

#20

Regarding hernias, which of the following is INCORRECT?

A. Umbilical hernias, when present at birth, usually obliterate by 2 years of age.

B. Femoral hernias often become incarcerated or strangulated because of the small defined space.

C. There is a type of hernia (Richter hernia) that can cause incarceration and strangulation without obstruction.

D. A Spigelian hernia occurs at the lateral edge of the rectus.

E. Once an incisional hernia is repaired, recurrence is rare.

#20

Answer: E

Incisional hernias occur after 2-10% of all abdominal operations secondary to breakdown of the fascial closure of prior surgery. Recurrence rates even after a repair can be as great as 45%.

1. **Indirect inguinal hernias** tract through the inguinal canal as a result of a persistent process vaginalis. The inguinal canal is located approximately midway between the pubic symphysis and the anterior iliac spine. The canal proceeds down along the inguinal ligament to the external ring, located medial to the inferior epigastric arteries.

2. **Direct inguinal hernias** usually occurs due to a defect or weakness in the transversalis fascia area of the Hesselbach triangle. The triangle is defined inferiorly by the inguinal ligament, laterally by the inferior epigastric arteries, and medially by the conjoined tendon.

3. **Femoral hernias** tract below the inguinal ligament through the femoral canal. The canal lies medial to the femoral vein. There is a greater risk of femoral hernia incarceration and strangulation compared to other hernia types.

4. **Umbilical hernias** occurs through the umbilical ring and usually closes by 2 years of age.

5. **Richter hernias** occur when a small portion of bowel herniates through a fascial defect. Obstruction is rare although incarceration and strangulation is common. The hernia can occur in almost any location and is usually related to prior laparoscopic procedures.

6. **Spigelian hernias** occur through a defect in the spigelian fascia, which is defined by the lateral edge of the rectus

muscle.

7. **Obturator hernias** pass through the obturator foramen, following the path of the obturator nerves and muscles. They are more common in females and commonly present with bowel obstructions.

- *Rutkow IM. The recurrence rate in hernia surgery. How important is it? Arch Surg. 1995 Jun; 130(6):575-6.*

#21

You have successfully performed a paracentesis on a patient who presents with increased abdominal girth and a new diagnosis of ascites. The serum-ascites albumin gradient is 2.0 g/dl. Which of the following diagnoses is LEAST likely to be the etiology of this patient's ascites?

A. Peritoneal carcinomatosis

B. Alcoholic hepatitis

C. Cardiac ascites

D. Portal vein thrombosis

E. Budd-Chiari syndrome

#21
Answer: A

The serum ascites albumin gradient is calculated by subtracting the albumin level in ascitic fluid from the serum albumin level. Values of 1.1 g/dL or greater indicate portal hypertension as the cause of the ascites with an accuracy of 97%. Values of less than 1.1 g/dL are indicative of other causes, such as peritoneal carcinomatosis, tuberculous peritonitis, pancreatic ascites, biliary ascites, nephrotic syndrome, or serositis.

- *Thomsen TW. Paracentesis. N Engl J Med. 2006 Nov 9; 355(19): e21.*
- *Hou W, Sanyal AJ. Ascites: diagnosis and management. Med Clin North Am. 2009 Jul; 93(4): 801-17*

#22

You are seeing a 75 year old male who comes in with bright red blood per rectum. He states that he has hemorrhoids and that when prolapse occurs, he must now manually reduce the hemorrhoids. He has already been taking sitz baths and drinking Metamucil and fiber supplements. What is the grade of his internal hemorrhoid and what is the best associated treatment?

A. I, excision

B. II, sitz baths

C. III, rubber band ligation

D. IV, hemorrhoidectomy

E. None of the above

#22

Answer: C

Internal hemorrhoids have been graded across a spectrum of severity, which has proven useful for guiding treatment options.

Grade I: The hemorrhoids do not prolapse.

Grade II: The hemorrhoids prolapse upon defecation but reduce spontaneously.

Grade III: The hemorrhoids prolapse upon defecation and must be reduced manually.

Grade IV: The hemorrhoids are prolapsed and cannot be reduced manually.

Surgical procedures can occur as an outpatient with the goal being removal of the excess hemorrhoidal tissue. Examples of these treatments include:

1. Rubber band ligation
2. Infrared coagulation
3. Bipolar diathermy (Bicap)
4. Laser photocoagulation
5. Sclerotherapy
6. Cryosurgery

Rubber band ligation first used in the 1960s is the most commonly used treatment in the U.S. for recurrent and symptomatic internal hemorrhoids. Grade I-III hemorrhoids are often treated with banding, which causes thrombosis followed by submucosal scarring.

Before outpatient intervention, diet control to reduce straining may prevent recurrence. Increasing fiber and water intake may be sufficient. Ice and topical analgesia can also relieve the pain of acute thrombosis.

- *Sneider EB, Maykel JA: Diagnosis and management of symptomatic hemorrhoids. Surg Clin North Am. 2010; 90: 17-32.*

#23

A healthy 50 year old male presents with severe abdominal pain for the past 2 days. He has severe nausea and vomiting and has been unable to eat food or drink water for 1 day. He is febrile with a temperature is 38.5°C and his heart rate is 120 beats per minute. On examination he is not peritoneal but has severe left lower quadrant abdominal pain. Which of the following is NOT indicated at this time in terms of management?

A. CT scan for diagnosis of diverticulitis and complications

B. Admission for IV fluid hydration, parenteral antibiotics, and nothing by mouth (NPO) status

C. Emergency colonoscopy

D. If CT scan demonstrates overt perforation, large abscess with gross peritoneal contamination, or obstruction then obtain a surgery consultation.

E. If CT scan demonstrates small perforation and small abscess collection (greater than 4 cm but without gross peritoneal contamination), percutaneous CT-guided drainage may be sufficient treatment.

#23

Answer: C

Colonoscopy and sigmoidoscopy are typically avoided when acute diverticulitis is suspected because of the risk of perforation or other exacerbation of the disease process. Expert opinion favors a cool-down period of 6 weeks.

This patient, however, requires IV hydration and admission due to his persistent vomiting. He requires broad-spectrum antibiotics (e.g., ciprofloxacin and metronidazole) and should remain NPO in case an emergent surgical procedure is needed and also to provide bowel rest.

CT scan of the abdomen in this patient will most likely demonstrate Hinchey stage 1 or 2 disease and he will probably be ready for discharge in 2-3 days. After resolution of symptoms as an outpatient he can have an elective colonoscopy. In general, less than 10% of patients admitted for diverticulitis require emergent surgical procedures.

The indications for emergency operative treatment include:

1. Peritonitis
2. Severe Sepsis
3. Uncontained perforations
4. The presence of a large, undrainable (inaccessible) abscess
5. Clinical deterioration within 3 days of medical management

Eligibility for percutaneous drainage will be based on the abscess size and location. Most patients with pericolic abscesses (< 4 cm) will have a good clinical course with bowel rest and broad spectrum antibiotics. Large abscess (> 4 cm) may be amenable to CT-guided percutaneous drainage.

- *Jacobs DO. Diverticulitis. N Engl J Med. 2007 Nov 15; 357(20): 2057-66. full text*

#24

You are seeing a patient who has undergone a Roux-en-Y gastric bypass 2 years ago and has sustained a 150 pound weight loss. In addition to all of the mechanical complications that may occur post-operatively, there are some nutritional deficiencies that can also result. Which of the following is NOT one of the nutritional deficiencies?

A. Vitamin C

B. Vitamin D

C. Vitamin B12

D. Iron

E. Calcium

#24

Answer: A

After undergoing Roux-en-Y, many patients will develop nutritional deficiencies in iron, vitamin B12, vitamin D, and calcium. Most patients have an uneventful course while receiving vitamin supplementation and frequent monitoring. Patients also develop secondary hyperparathyroidism after Roux-en-Y. They experience increased bone turnover and decreased bone density. The consequences of bone density loss manifest most in postmenopausal women.

- *Edwards ED, et al. Presentation and management of common post-weight loss surgery problems in the emergency department. Ann Emerg Med. 2006; 47: 160-166. full text*

#25

Early major complications after a Roux-en-Y gastric by-pass include all of the following EXCEPT:

A. Internal hernia

B. Anastomotic leak

C. Intra-abdominal bleeding

D. Pulmonary embolism

E. Deep vein thrombosis

#25

Answer: A

Early major complications include anastomotic leak, bleeding, thrombosis (DVT or PE). Internal hernias occur later in the clinical course if they were to develop. The following table highlights common complications in Roux-en-Y gastric bypass patients:

Complication	Presentation	Diagnosis	Management
Stricture/stenosis	Inability to tolerate oral intake, dysphagia	UGI series, upper endoscopy	Endoscopic dilatation
Marginal ulcer	Epigastric abdominal pain, dyspepsia	Upper endoscopy	Acid suppression therapy
Internal hernia	Intermittent, crampy abdominal pain	CT scan, UGI series	Surgical consultation
Reflux	Dyspepsia, new-onset asthma/worsening preexisting pulmonary disease	Upper endoscopy, cholescintigraphy	Acid suppression therapy, surgical consultation
Nutritional	Anemia, neuropathy, fractures, hypercalcemia	CBC	B12 and iron supplementation

- *Edwards ED, et al. Presentation and management of common post-weight loss surgery problems in the emergency department. Ann Emerg Med. 2006 Feb; 47(2): 160-6. full text*

#26

You are seeing a patient in whom you suspect cholecystitis. True statements about this disease process include all of the following EXCEPT:

(Choose two answers.)

A. Jaundice is commonly seen with cholecystitis

B. Risk factors for biliary colic and cholecystitis include pregnancy, elderly population, obesity, certain ethnic groups, and drugs.

C. Risk factors for acalculous cholecystitis include diabetes, HIV, vascular disease, total parenteral nutrition, prolonged fasting, or being an ICU patient.

D. Peritoneal signs are seen in up to 95% of patients with cholecystitis.

E. Ultrasonography and nuclear medicine studies are the best imaging studies for the diagnosis of both cholecystitis and cholelithiasis.

#26

Answers: A and D

Jaundice is unusual in the early stages of acute cholecystitis and may be found in fewer than 20% of patients. Jaundice should raise suspicion of choledocholithiasis, Mirizzi's syndrome (obstruction of the bile duct as a result of external compression of a stone in the gallbladder or cystic duct), and cholangitis. Most patients with uncomplicated cholecystitis do not have peritoneal signs, and if they do, be suspicious for emphysematous cholecystitis, gangrenous cholecystitis, or perforation. The other statements are true.

- *Strasberg S. Acute Calculous Cholecystitis. N Engl J Med. 2008 Jun 26; 358(26): 2804-11. full text*

#27

You are seeing a patient with pancreatitis at a community hospital. A surgical consult may be indicated in which of the following scenarios?

A. Pancreatic phlegmon seen on CT

B. Hemorrhagic pancreatitis seen on CT

C. Gallstone pancreatitis in which a sphincterotomy has already been performed

D. No improvement despite interventional radiology-guided drainage of necrotic pancreatitis

E. All of the above

#27

Answer: E

Consideration for consulting a surgeon should be made in the following cases:

1. Hemorrhagic pancreatitis, since surgery may be required to achieve hemostasis.
2. Patients who fail to improve despite optimal medical treatment.
3. Biliary pancreatitis, as a sphincterotomy and cholecystectomy can relieve the obstruction and prevent recurrence.

- *McFadden DW, Reber HA. Indications for surgery in severe acute pancreatitis. Int J Pancreatol. 1994 Apr; 15(2): 83-90.*

#28

You are seeing a patient in whom you suspect pancreatitis. True statements about this disease process include all of the following EXCEPT:

(Choose two answers.)

A. ARDS, acute renal failure, cardiac depression, hemorrhage, and hypotensive shock all may be systemic manifestations of acute pancreatitis in its most severe form.

B. The major causes are long-standing alcohol consumption and gallstones.

C. CT is the most reliable imaging modality in the diagnosis of acute pancreatitis.

D. Antibiotic coverage of enterococcal species is indicated in simple pancreatitis.

E. Nasogastric (NG) tube should be inserted in all cases.

#28

Answers: D and E

Antibiotics are not routinely indicated for uncomplicated pancreatitis. However, when you suspect a phlegmon, cholangitis, or septic shock as a result of the pancreatitis, broad spectrum antibiotics are indicated. The preferred antibiotics provide coverage for organisms for the biliary system, such as ampicillin and third-generation cephalosporins. If the patient is not obstructed, an NG tube is not necessary.

- *Whitcomb D. Acute Pancreatitis. N Engl J Med. 2006 May 18; 354(20): 2142-50.*

#29

A patient presents with dysphagia and odynophagia while eating a heavy holiday meal. She begins to not tolerate her own salivary secretions and believes that she has a food impaction. Which of the following is NOT appropriate for management?

A. Beta-blocker

B. Soft-tissue lateral neck X-ray, chest X-ray and KUB X-ray

C. Glucagon

D. Calling in gastroenterology

E. Motility studies may be warranted as an outpatient.

#29

Answer: A

A food bolus usually consists of meat lodged at or above a stricture or ring. Patients with total obstruction require immediate intervention. Endoscopy can be deferred in patients in whom the food bolus impaction resolves spontaneously. However, endoscopy, biopsy, and in some cases esophageal motility studies should be performed at some later date because of the high likelihood of underlying esophageal structural or motor abnormality. Gastroenterologists will frequently perform a dilation after identification of the esophageal stricture.

In an acute impaction which has not passed spontaneously, the endoscopist can first attempt to push the bolus into the stomach with the distal tip of the endoscope. Besides stricture, eosinophilic esophagitis (EE) is also a common cause of food impaction.

Administration of glucagon (1.0 mg IV) can be attempted to relax the esophagus, which may promote passage of the food bolus. Patients should be given an antiemetic prior to administration of glucagon.

- *Leopard D, Fishpool S, Winter S. The management of oesophageal soft food bolus obstruction: a systematic review. Ann R Coll Surg Engl. Sep 2011; 93(6): 441-4. full text*

- *Al-Haddad M, et al. Glucagon for the relief of esophageal food impaction does it really work? Dig Dis Sci. 2006 Nov; 51(11): 1930-3.*

#30

You are caring for a patient with chronic hepatic failure, and you are speaking to a hepatologist at a tertiary hospital. He asks you to calculate the MELD (model for end-stage liver disease) score. Components of the MELD include which of the following?

(Choose three answers.)

A. ALT

B. Albumin

C. INR

D. Creatinine

E. Bilirubin

#30

Answer: C, D, and E

MELD is a prospectively developed and validated chronic liver disease severity scoring system that uses a patient's laboratory values for serum bilirubin, serum creatinine, and the INR to predict survival. The MELD score, as currently used by UNOS in prioritizing allocation of organs for liver transplantation, is calculated according to the following formula:

MELD = 3.8[Ln serum bilirubin (mg/dL)] + 11.2[Ln INR] + 9.6[Ln serum creatinine (mg/dL)] + 6.4

The MELD score also has prognostic value in several clinical settings outside of liver transplantation, including predicting mortality associated with: alcoholic hepatitis, hepatorenal syndrome, fulminant hepatic failure, sepsis in cirrhosis, acute variceal hemorrhage, surgical procedures in chronic liver disease patients, and the TIPS procedure.

- *Kamath PS, Kim WR, Advanced Liver Disease Study Group. The model for end-stage liver disease (MELD). Hepatology. 2007 Mar; 45(3): 797-805.*
- *MD Calc -MELD Score http://www.mdcalc.com/meld-score-model-for-end-stage-liver-disease-12-and-older/*

#31

The same hepatologist also asks you about his Modified Child-Turcotte-Pugh (CTP) Score. Which of the following is NOT a component of the CTP?

A. Albumin

B. Presence of ascites

C. Presence of encephalopathy

D. Presence of varices

E. Bilirubin

#31

Answer: D

The current CTP scoring system is based upon five parameters: serum bilirubin, serum albumin, prothrombin time, ascites and encephalopathy and nutritional status. It was then modified to include INR (Modified Child-Pugh classification). In general, the MELD score is more widely used and standardized.

.*Angermayr B, et al. Child-Pugh versus MELD score in predicting survival in patients undergoing transjugular intrahepatic portosystemic shunt. Gut. 2003 Jun; 52(6): 879-85.*

. *MD Calc http://www.mdcalc.com/child-pugh-score-for-cirrhosis-mortality/*

#32

You are seeing a patient with an anorectal foreign body. Which of the following are contraindications to attempted removal in the ED and an indication for surgical consultation?

A. Signs of perforation, obstruction, or severe abdominal pain

B. If the foreign body is nonpalpable

C. If there is broken glass in the rectum

D. If the patient is uncooperative or intolerant of attempts to examination

E. All of the above

#32

Answer: E

The indications for bedside anorectal foreign body removal:

1. Patient is stable and cooperative
2. Foreign body is palpable by rectal approach
3. Foreign body is without sharp edges or broken glass

Surgical consultation should be obtained immediately if:

1. The patient has signs of perforation, obstruction, or peritonitis
2. If it is a nonpalpable foreign body
3. If there is broken glass
4. If the patient is uncooperative or intolerant of the exam in the ED
5. If you do not have the equipment necessary for retrieval

- *Koornstra JJ, Weersma RK. Management of rectal foreign bodies: description of a new technique and clinical practice guidelines. World J Gastroenterol. Jul 21 2008; 14(27): 4403-6. full text*

#33

You are treating a patient with diverticulitis complicated by fistula formation. Regarding this entity, which of the following is TRUE?

A. The major types of fistulas are colovesical fistulas, and colovaginal fistulas.

B. Common symptoms with a colovesical fistula include pneumaturia, dysuria, or irritative symptoms, and fecaluria.

C. Computed tomography (CT), barium enema (BE), colonoscopy, cystoscopy, and intravenous urography (IVU) can all diagnose a colovesical fistula.

D. CT diagnosis is usually made by the combination of local colonic thickening adjacent to an area of thickened bladder, associated diverticula, and oral contrast material or air in the bladder.

E. All of the above

#33

Answer: E

Fistula formation is one of the complications of diverticulitis, accounting for up to 20% of surgically treated cases of diverticular disease. In western countries diverticulitis usually involves the sigmoid colon.

The major fistulas are:

1. Colovesical
2. Colovaginal
3. Coloenteric
4. Colouterine.

In theory, a fistula can create a tract to any adjacent organ. Diverticulitis is the most common cause of a colovesical fistula, accounting for 40 to 90% of cases. CT, barium enema (BE), colonoscopy, cystoscopy, and intravenous urography are all useful modalities depending on the location of the fistula. Air within organs other than the bowel is highly suggestive of fistulization, making CT the initial modality of choice. CT can also assess for adjacent abscesses.

- *Rosen's Emergency Medicine - Concepts and Clinical Practice. 8th edition. 2013. Chapter 95: Disorders of the Large Intestine. 1262-1265.*

#34

You are seeing a patient with an external hemorrhoid that is thrombosed and painful. Which of the following are relative contraindications to excision of an acutely thrombosed external hemorrhoid?

A. If the patient presents after 72 hours of thrombosis

B. If the patient has Crohn's disease

C. If the patient is not in pain

D. Uncooperative patient

E. If the thrombosed hemorrhoid occurs in pregnant women

F. All of the above

#34

Answer: F

After 72 hours, most patients have decreased pain and spontaneous resolution of their acute thrombosis, and therefore excision is not indicated. Relative contraindications include Crohn's disease, since referral to a specialist may be preferred as there is a high rate of fistula formation. With pregnant women, most cases can be managed with Sitz baths, increased fiber, and PO fluids. Excision is usually necessary only for severe pain, as most hemorrhoids resolve after delivery. Uncooperative patients are best managed in the operating room.

- *Wolff BG, et al. The ASCRS Textbook of Colon and Rectal Surgery. 2007. Chapter 11. Springer Science and Business Media, LLC.*

#35

Regarding clostridium difficile colitis, which of the following statements is TRUE?

(Choose two answers.)

A. The overall incidence of C. difficile has declined over the last several years.

B. The overall virulence of C. difficile has declined over the last several years.

C. Toxins D and E are the main virulence determinants of C. diff.

D. Effective therapy is with either metronidazole or oral vancomycin.

E. Markers of severe C. difficile infection include pseudomembranous colitis, a marked peripheral leukocytosis, acute renal failure, and hypotension.

#35
Answer: D and E

During the mid- and late 1990s, the incidence of C. difficile infection in acute care hospitals was 30-40 cases per 100,000. Three bacterial factors have been implicated in outbreaks of C. difficile infection caused by the virulent NAP-1/027 strain:

1. Increased production of toxins A and B
2. Fluoroquinolone resistance
3. Production of binary toxin.

Toxins A and B determine the pathogenesis of C. difficile. There are non-toxin producing strains, as well. Despite the dramatic increases in the incidence and severity of the disease, oral vancomycin or IV or oral metronidazole remain effective treatments.

Pseudomembranous colitis, elevated peripheral leukocytosis, renal failure, and hypotension are poor prognostic signs for C. difficile infection and warrant aggressive supportive care and antibiotic therapy. In patients with obstruction, ileus or toxic megacolon, intravenous metronidazole (500 mg four times daily) should be used instead of oral vancomycin.

- *Kelly CP, Lamont JT. Clostridium difficile—more difficult than ever. N Engl J Med. 2008 Oct 30; 359(18):1932-40. full text*

#36

Regarding C. difficile infection, which of the following statements is TRUE?

A. The resistance rates to vancomycin are rising rapidly.

B. Recurrence of an infection usually occurs because of resistance to the antibiotic regimen (metronidazole or vancomycin).

C. Both of the above

D. Neither of the above

#36

Answer: D

Despite effective treatment with vancomycin and metronidazole, C. difficile recurrence remains common with rates as high as 20%. Fortunately, resistance to vancomycin and metronidazole is rare.

- *Kelly CP, Lamont JT. Clostridium difficile—more difficult than ever. N Engl J Med. 2008 Oct 30; 359(18):1932-40. full text*

#37

You are seeing a 7 year old child with abdominal pain and fever. You recall a JAMA article stating that fever is the single most useful sign associated with appendicitis as it increases the likelihood of appendicitis by 3.4 (95%CI 2.4-4.8) and its absence decreases the likelihood by 0.32 (95%CI 0.16-0.64). Which of the following increases the odds ratio for appendicitis the greatest, after presence of fever?

A. Rebound tenderness

B. Midabdominal pain migrating to the right lower quadrant

C. RLQ tenderness to palpation

D. WBC > 10,000 /mm^3

E. Age < 2 yo

#37

Answer: A

In children with abdominal pain, fever was the single most useful sign associated with appendicitis; a fever increases the likelihood of appendicitis (likelihood ratio [LR], 3.4; 95% confidence interval [CI], 2.4-4.8) and conversely, its absence decreases the chance of appendicitis (LR, 0.32; 95% CI, 0.16-0.64).

Rebound tenderness triples the odds of appendicitis (summary LR, 3.0; 95% CI, 2.3-3.9), while its absence reduces the likelihood (summary LR, 0.28; 95% CI, 0.14-0.55).

Midabdominal pain migrating to the right lower quadrant (LR range, 1.9-3.1) increases the risk of appendicitis more than right lower quadrant pain itself (summary LR, 1.2; 95% CI, 1.0-1.5).

A white blood cell count of less than 10,000/microL decreases the likelihood of appendicitis (summary LR, 0.22; 95% CI, 0.17-0.30), as does an absolute neutrophil count of 6750/microL or lower (LR, 0.06; 95% CI, 0.03-0.16). Symptoms and signs are most useful in combination, particularly for identifying children who do not require further evaluation or intervention.

- *Bundy DG, et al. Does this child have appendicitis? JAMA. July 2007; 298(4): 438-451. full text*

#38

Which of the following is an indication for operative management in acute diverticulitis?

(Choose two answers.)

A. Fever greater than 40.0ºC

B. Leukocytosis > 16,000 /mm^3

C. Generalized peritonitis

D. Undrainable (inaccessible abscess)

E. Neutrophils greater than 85%

#38

Answer: C and D

Some patients admitted for acute diverticulitis undergo surgical intervention. Determination of the need for surgery is multifactorial, with the severity of the disease and comorbidities playing the greatest role. In general, surgical indications are peritonitis, uncontrolled sepsis, uncontained visceral perforation, the presence of a large, undrainable (inaccessible) abscess, and lack of improvement or deterioration despite 3 days of medical management.

- *Jacobs DO. Diverticulitis. N Engl J Med. 2007 Nov 15; 357(20): 2057-66.*

#39

You are about to do a paracentesis on a patient with a history of multiple abdominal surgeries. What adjunct can help you reduce the risk of iatrogenic injury in this patient?

A. Use of ultrasound-guidance

B. Urethral catheterization

C. Nasogastric suction

D. Going through the surgical scar

E. Passing the catheter through visibly engorged cutaneous vessels

#39

Answer: A

Paracentesis should be performed with caution in pregnant patients or in patients who have organomegaly, bowel obstruction, intraabdominal adhesions, or a distended urinary bladder. The use of ultrasonographic guidance in these situations may reduce the risk of injury. Nasogastric decompression should only be considered before paracentesis in patients with bowel obstructions. Patients should be encouraged to empty their bladder. If urinary retention is present, then urethral catheterization is an option. The paracentesis catheter should not be passed through sites of cutaneous infection, visibly engorged cutaneous vessels, surgical scars, or abdominal wall hematomas.

- *Thomsen TW, et al. Paracentesis. N Engl J Med. 2006 Nov 9; 355(19): e21*

#40

You are seeing a 35 year old female who underwent a Roux-en-Y gastric bypass 1 week ago, and she is febrile and tachycardic but has no abdominal pain. She has a benign abdomen on examination. The chest X-ray and the urinalysis are negative. What is the most likely etiology of the fever and the tachycardia?

A. Deep vein thrombosis

B. Intra-abdominal bleeding

C. Bowel obstruction

D. Adhesions

E. Anastomotic leak

#40

Answer: E

Early major complications include anastomotic leak, intra-abdominal bleeding, and deep venous thrombosis or pulmonary embolism. Any patient who presents in the first weeks after a Roux-en-Y with tachycardia and fever might be harboring an anastomotic leak with associated abscess. The physical examination in the morbidly obese is difficult. Any remote suspicion for an intra-abdominal process, especially in a patient who recently underwent a gastric bypass, should trigger ordering of a CT scan of the abdomen and pelvis with oral and IV contrast.

- *Edwards ED, et al. Presentation and Management of Common Post-weight loss surgery problems in the Emergency Department. Annals of Emerg Med. 2006; 47: 160-166. full text*

#41

You are seeing a patient who underwent the LAP-band procedure 2 months ago, and she is unable to tolerate anything by mouth because of intractable vomiting. What should be done?

A. Intravenous hydration

B. The lap-band should be deflated as quickly as possible.

C. Prompt surgical consultation

D. After the band is deflated, a water-soluble contrast swallow should be obtained.

E. All of the above

#41

Answer: E

Patients who present to the ED with a clinical diagnosis consistent with acute gastroesophageal obstruction and LAP-banding should have the band deflated in consultation with the surgeon. Deflation can prevent progression of the obstruction to gastric perforation. While stabilizing the band port with two fingers, infiltrate the overlying skin with lidocaine and then access the port with an 18 gauge needle. The standard reservoir holds 5 ml of saline. Fluoroscopy-guided deflation is also an option, if the reservoir is not accessible due to the patient's body habitus.

After band deflation, perform a water-soluble contrast swallow study. As stated above, prompt surgical consultation is warranted.

- *Edwards ED, et al. Presentation and Management of Common Post-weight loss surgery problems in the Emergency Department. Annals of Emerg Med. 2006; 47: 160-166. full text*

- *Bewsher SM, Azzi A, Wright T. Use of standard hypodermic needles for accessing laparoscopic adjustable gastric band ports. Obes Surg. 2010 Jun; 20(6): 761-7.*

#42

The two predominant viruses that have been implicated in causing gastroenteritis in the United States are:

(Choose two answers.)

A. Coronavirus

B. Norovirus

C. Calicivirus

D. Rotavirus

E. Parvovirus

#42

Answer: B and D

Viral gastroenteritis is the second leading cause of illness in the United States. Although several virus families have been implicated, including caliciviruses, corona viruses, and parvoviruses, norovirus and rotavirus predominate.

- *Payne D, et al. Norovirus and Medically Attended Gastroenteritis in U.S. Children. N Engl J Med. 2013 Mar 21; 368(12): 1121-30.*

#43

TRUE statements about the focused abdominal sonography in trauma (FAST US include which of the following:

A. FAST can image diaphragmatic defects well.

B. FAST can image the retroperitoneum well.

C. FAST can detect sensitively detect 500 mL of fluid.

D. FAST has a 100% sensitivity in detecting as little as 100 ml of intraperitoneal fluid.

E. All of the above

#43
Answer: C

The FAST US has a sensitivity in detecting as little as 100 mL and more typically 500 mL of intraperitoneal fluid, and ranges from 60 to 95% sensitivity in most studies. The FAST does not image the retroperitoneum, or diaphragmatic injuries well. Its sensitivity can be limited by obesity, excessive bowel gas or subcutaneous air. Note that it cannot distinguish blood from ascites, and US has a high false negative rate in detecting hemoperitoneum in the presence of a pelvic fracture.

- *Tsui C, et al. Focused abdominal sonography for trauma in the emergency department for blunt abdominal trauma. Int J Emerg Med. Sep 2008; 1(3): 183–187. full text*

#44

Possible etiologies of encephalopathy in a known cirrhotic patient include which of the following?

(Choose three answers.)

A. Hyperkalemia

B. Acidosis

C. Hypokalemia

D. Alkalosis

E. GI bleeding

#44

Answer: C, D, and E

Hypokalemia, alkalosis, and GI bleeding contribute to increased ammonia production or decreased absorption. Altered mental status in a cirrhotic can also be caused by hyponatremia, hypoglycemia, azotemia, sepsis, and dehydration.

- *Rosen's Emergency Medicine - Concepts and Clinical Practice. 8th edition. 2013. Chapter 90: Disorders of the Liver and Biliary Tree. 1194-1195.*

#45

TRUE statements about peritonitis in patients on peritoneal dialysis (PD) include which of the following?

A. The majority of the cases of peritonitis are caused by gram negative enteric organisms.

B. Diagnosis is often made by the patient when a cloudy dialysis effluent is noted.

C. Diagnosis is confirmed in the ED by finding more than 500 WBCs/mm in the peritoneal fluid, with more than 250 PMNs.

D. PD-associated peritonitis usually has to be treated with intravenous antibiotics.

E. None of the above

#45

Answer: B

Peritonitis in patients on PD is caused by bacterial contamination of the dialysate or tubing during an exchange. The majority of the cases are caused by Staph aureus or Staph epidermidis, while 20% may be due to gram negative enteric organisms. The disease differs from spontaneous bacterial peritonitis where most bacteria are gram negative organisms. The diagnosis is often made by the patient when a cloudy dialysis effluent is noted, and it is often accompanied by nonspecific abdominal pain, malaise, or fever.

The diagnosis of PD-peritonitis is confirmed by the finding of more than 100 WBC/mm in the peritoneal fluid, with more than 50% neutrophils, or by a positive gram stain. PD-associated peritonitis usually can be treated with an initial intraperitoneal loading dose of antibiotic, followed by a 10 to 14 day course of intraperitoneal antibiotics, often administered on an outpatient basis. Obviously, patients who have severe abdominal pain, vomiting, or hypotension should be hospitalized.

- *Rosen's Emergency Medicine - Concepts and Clinical Practice. 8th edition. 2013. Chapter 97: Renal Failure. 1310-1311.*

#46

It is Thanksgiving Day, and you are the ED physician on when a 55 yo male comes in complaining of "a piece of turkey stuck in my throat." He appears to be having difficulty with his secretions, as he continues to spit out his saliva and drools intermittently. He is not hoarse, and this has never happened to him before. While you are seeing two other patients he fortunately passes the piece of meat and is no longer spitting or drooling. What is your next best step?

A. Discharge him to home without any follow-up, as he is your one "cure" tonight.

B. Discharge him to home without any follow-up with a liquid diet.

C. Arrange a follow-up endoscopy .

D. Admit the patient for observation.

E. Order an ECG as this could be his anginal equivalent.

#46

Answer: C

Endoscopy is indicated in all patients suffering from food impaction, whether the food bolus is eventually passed or not. Food impaction may be the first sign of an obstructive lesion.

. *Roberts and Hedges' Clinical Procedures in Emergency Medicine. 6th edition. 2013. Chapter 39: Esophageal Foreign Bodies. 789-808.*

#47

You are seeing a patient who presents with an episode of syncope following several weeks of fatigue. His blood pressure is 90/60 mm Hg, pulse is 105 bpm, and black, foul smelling stool is found on rectal examination. His hemoglobin is 6.5 mg/dL. Which of the following factors increase the likelihood of an upper GI bleed?

(Choose two answers.)

A. Blood clots in the stool

B. Melena

C. Serum urea nitrogen to creatinine ratio of 15:1

D. Hemoglobin of 10 mg/dL

E. Nasogastric lavage with blood

#47

Answer: B and E

Melena, NG lavage with blood or coffee grounds, or BUN/Cr ratio of > 30 increase the likelihood of a upper GI bleed. Blood clots in the stool make a UGIB much less likely. However all of these tests and findings should be taken in the clinical context of the patient.

Regarding the nasogastric tube, patients rate it as one of the most painful procedures. There is questionable efficacy of the procedure helping to differentiate an upper GI bleed from a lower GI bleed.

- *Srygley FD, et al. Does this patient have a severe upper gastrointestinal bleed? JAMA. 2012; 307: 1072-1079. full text*

#48

Which of the following factors increase the likelihood for a SEVERE upper GI bleed?

(Choose two answers.)

A. Hemoglobin < 8 g/dL

B. BUN > 90 mg/dL

C. SBP of 120 mm Hg

D. Pulse rate of 95 bpm

E. History of diabetes

#48

Answer: A and B

A hemoglobin of < 8 mg/dL, a BUN > 90 mg/dL , WBC > 12k $/mm^3$ all increase the likelihood of a severe UGI bleed.

The Blatchford score can identify patients with a low likelihood of a severe GI bleed. The criteria include:

1. BUN
2. Hemoglobin
3. Systolic blood pressure
4. Heart rate
5. Presentation with melena or syncope
6. Underlying hepatic disease
7. CHF

Note that the Blatchford score does not require an NG lavage.

- *Srygley FD, et al. Does this patient have a severe upper gastrointestinal bleed? JAMA. 2012; 307: 1072-1079. full text*
- *MDCalc - Blatchford Score http://www.mdcalc.com/glasgow-blatchford-bleeding-score-gbs/*

#49

Which of the following is the single most useful sign associated with appendicitis in children who present with abdominal pain?

A. Anorexia

B. Nausea/Vomiting

C. Right lower quadrant tenderness

D. Fever

E. Diarrhea

#49

Answer: D

In children with abdominal pain, fever was the most useful sign associated with appendicitis. A fever increases the likelihood of appendicitis (likelihood ratio [LR], 3.4; 95% CI, 2.4-4.8) and, its absence decreases the chance of appendicitis (LR, 0.32; 95% CI, 0.16-0.64).

In children with suspected appendicitis, rebound tenderness triples the odds of appendicitis (LR, 3.0; 95% CI, 2.3-3.9), while its absence reduces the likelihood (LR, 0.28; 95% CI, 0.14-0.55).

Midabdominal pain migrating to the right lower quadrant (LR range, 1.9-3.1) increases the risk of appendicitis more than right lower quadrant pain itself (LR, 1.2; 95% CI, 1.0-1.5)

A white blood cell count of less than 10,000/mm^3 decreases the likelihood of appendicitis (LR, 0.22; 95% CI, 0.17-0.30). An absolute neutrophil count less than 6750/mm3 or lower (LR, 0.06; 95% CI, 0.03-0.16) also decreases the likelihood of appendicitis. Symptoms and signs are most useful in combination, particularly for identifying children who do not require further evaluation or intervention.

- *Bundy DG, et al. Does this child have appendicitis? JAMA. 2007 Jul 25; 298(4): 438-51. full text*

HEMATOLOGY

#1

Regarding a patient with Thrombotic Thrombocytopenic Purpura (TTP) and Hemolytic Uremic Syndrome (HUS), which of the following statements is FALSE?

A. TTP and adult HUS are clinically similar disorders that present with microangiopathic hemolytic anemia and thrombocytopenia.

B. Platelet transfusions are the treatment of choice for TTP.

C. TTP is more common in the adults and HUS is more common in pediatrics.

D. E. coli O157:H7 is recognized as the leading cause of HUS in the United States, Canada, and Europe.

E. Although the pentad of symptoms and laboratory findings is described classically in TTP, only 40% of patients manifest all five criteria.

#1

Answer: B

Despite significant thrombocytopenia and clinical bleeding, platelet transfusions are contraindicated in TTP. More thrombi are formed in the tissues when additional platelets are supplied. The mainstay of current therapy for TTP is plasma exchange with fresh frozen plasma (plasmapheresis). Prednisone, in doses of 1mg/kg/d is often given, but the mainstay of treatment is plasma exchange. Other than E. coli 0157:H7, HIV infection, chemotherapeutic agents, and radiation therapy have been reported to be associated with HUS. All of the other statements are true.

- *Zhou A, Mehta RS, Smith RE. Outcomes of platelet transfusion in patients with thrombotic thrombocytopenic purpura: a retrospective case series study. Ann Hematol. 2015 Mar; 94(3): 467-72.*

#2

Regarding sickle cell disease, which of the following statements is FALSE?

A. Painful vaso-occlusive events are the most common presenting problem for sickle cell patients in the emergency department.

B. Hemolytic crisis is the leading cause of death in the sickle cell patient.

C. Evaluate for evidence of an acute infection precipitating the vaso-occlusive crisis.

D. Most sickle cell patients have a persistent mild leukocytosis and a moderate anemia (hematocrit of 20-30%).

#2

Answer: B

Hemolytic crisis can occur during a vaso-occlusive episode when large numbers of sickled cells occlude the vasculature. Splenic sequestration crisis can lead to splenic infarctions, anemia and hypotension. Infection is the leading overall cause of morbidity in patients with sickle cell disease. Acute Chest Syndrome (ACS) is the leading cause of death. Patients with ACS present similarly to those with pneumonia and have fever, chest pain, cough, hypoxia, and a new infiltrate on chest X-ray. Common infectious causes are Chlamydia, Mycoplasma, and RSV. ACS also involves pulmonary microvascular sludging and infarction. All of the other statements are true.

- *Steinberg, M. Management of Sickle Cell Disease. N Engl J Med. 1999 Apr 1; 340(13): 1021-30. full text*

#3

A 24 year old male (weight of 80 kg) with severe Hemophilia A (factor 8 deficiency with level of 1% with no inhibitors) is brought in by paramedics after he sustains a fall and a head injury. The patient appears to be confused and has a hematoma to his occiput and multiple abrasions. What is the most important next step in management?

A. Obtain a Head CT

B. Obtain a diffusion-perfusion MRI of his head

C. Transfuse DDAVP

D. Calculate amount of factor 8 needed – 3960 units - and begin immediate transfusion

E. Calculate amount of factor 8 needed – 7920 units - and begin immediate transfusion

#3

Answer: D

Diagnostic tests should not delay initiation of treatment with factor 8. The number of units of factor 8 needed equals:

(weight in kg) x (50ml plasma/kg) x (1 unit factor VIII/ml plasma) x (desired factor 8 level – native factor 8 level) = 80 x 50 x 1x 0.99 = 3960 units

Half this dose should be readministered in 12 hours.

DDAVP can also be used (it raises factor 8 levels) as a supplement, and antifibrinolytics may also be helpful, especially in mucosal bleeds.

With factor 9 deficiency, the "50ml plasma/kg" is replaced by "100 ml plasma/kg," and thus the required dose is doubled (the volume of distribution of factor VIII is 50ml/kg, whereas the volume of distribution of factor IX is 100ml/kg). Because factor IX has a longer half-life, the repeated dose does not need to be administered until 24 hours after the first dose. DDAVP is not helpful for those with factor 9 deficiency, since it does not raise factor 9 levels.

- *Singleton T, Kruse-Jarres R, Leissinger C. Emergency department care for patients with hemophilia and von Willebrand disease. J Emerg Med. 2010 Aug; 39(2): 158-65.*

#4

Regarding drug-induced thrombocytopenia, which of the following statements is FALSE?

A. Heparin-induced thrombocytopenia is the most common drug-related cause of a drop in the platelet count, but thrombosis, rather than thrombocytopenia, more commonly occurs.

B. Severely affected patients have purpura and bleeding from the nose, gums, and gastrointestinal or urinary tract and thrombocytopenia is often <20,000 platelets/mm^3.

C. Typically, a patient will have used a drug for > 1 week before presenting with thrombocytopenia.

D. Corticosteroids are the treatment of choice.

E. Drug sensitivity probably persists indefinitely

#4

Answer: D

Many patients with drug-induced thrombocytopenia have only petechial hemorrhages and occasional ecchymoses and often require no specific treatment other than discontinuation of the sensitizing medication. When there is uncertainty about the causative drug, all medications should be discontinued, and equivalents with different chemical structures can be tried as substitutes. Patients who have active bleeding should be aggressively treated with platelet transfusions because of the risk of fatal intracranial or intrapulmonary hemorrhage. Corticosteroids are often given, but there is little evidence that they are helpful for drug-induced causes. Intravenous immune globulin and plasma exchange have been used in acutely ill patients, but the benefits are also uncertain.

Once established, drug sensitivity should be assumed to persist indefinitely, and patients should be advised to avoid the medication.

- *Aster RH, et al. Drug-induced immune thrombocytopenia. N Engl J Med. 2007 Aug 9; 357(6): 580-7. full text*

#5

Regarding disseminated intravascular coagulation (DIC), which of the following is FALSE?

A. DIC occurs in an acute form and a chronic form.

B. The acute form is usually associated with sepsis, trauma, transfusion reactions, and acute obstetric events.

C. Hypertension is a common presentation in the acute form of DIC.

D. Thrombosis can also occur in association with bleeding.

E. Patients present with acute bleeding from multiple sites.

#5

Answer: C

Patients with acute DIC often present with fever, overt bleeding, and hypotension. Signs of thromboses are often subtle and manifest as abnormal mental status, dyspnea, abdominal pain, deteriorating renal function, acral cyanosis, and gangrene. There is often bleeding and thrombosis with intravascular deposition of fibrin causing microthrombi, which then leads to organ failure.

- *Levi M, Ten Cate H. Disseminated intravascular coagulation. N Engl J Med. Aug 19 1999; 341(8): 586-92. full text*

#6

Which of the following statements about idiopathic thrombocytopenic purpura is TRUE?

A. Patients may present with petechiae.

B. Significant bleeding is rare.

C. The mainstay of treatment is platelet repletion with a transfusion.

D. In most children, ITP resolves spontaneously and does not recur.

E. A, B, and D.

#6

Answer: E

Most cases of ITP resolve spontaneously and never need intervention. If the platelet count is less than 10,000, treatment with IVIG should be considered, and the dose may be repeated after 24 hours. A response should be expected in 24 to 48 hours. Other treatment options include steroids, plasmapheresis, rituximab, and other chemotherapeutics. Platelet transfusions should be avoided unless there is life threatening active bleeding, since the underlying immune process will further destroy the transfused platelets.

- *Sandler SG, Tutuncuoglu SO. Immune thrombocytopenic purpura - current management practices. Expert Opin Pharmacother. 2004; 5(12): 2515-27.*

#7

You are seeing a patient who presents with petechial hemorrhages after beginning TMP-SMX 7 days ago and quinine yesterday. You find on laboratory examination that she has a platelet count of 10. Which of the following is the most likely etiology of the thrombocytopenia?

A. TMP-SMX

B. Quinine

C. Neither

D. Both

#7

Answer: A

In drug-induced thrombocytopenia, the effect occurs over 5-7 days as sensitization takes place. In this case the 1 day of quinine is most likely not contributing to the thrombocytopenia but if the time course was vague all medications should be discontinued. The drug induced antibodies are specific to the sensitizing drug, so a drug in a similar class can be attempted with close monitoring in the future.

- *Aster RH, et al. Drug-induced thrombocytopenia. N Engl J Med. 2007 Aug 9; 357(6): 580-7. full text*

#8

You are seeing a patient in whom you suspect tumor lysis syndrome (TLS). Which of the following laboratory abnormalities would NOT be expected?

A. Hyperkalemia

B. Hypercalcemia

C. Hypocalcemia

D. Uric acid elevation

E. Hyperphosphatemia

#8

Answer: B

Laboratory studies usually show elevated uric acid, phosphorus, potassium, and lactate dehydrogenase levels and a low calcium level. Every attempt should be made to anticipate and prevent TLS in patients at risk. The risk of TLS can be reduced by administering allopurinol for 2 to 3 days before planned chemotherapy and by maintaining good hydration status.

Patients at high risk with a large tumor burden may benefit from intravenous recombinant urate oxidase (rasburicase). Aggressive treatment of hyperkalemia is indicated. Diuretics such as furosemide can be used cautiously to increase urine output if the patient is not hypovolemic. Hyperphosphatemia can be treated with phosphate binders. Dialysis is indicated in renal failure, congestive heart failure, or severe hyperkalemia or patients who do not respond to medical therapy. Hypocalcemia should not be treated unless symptomatic.

- *Halfdanarson TR, et al. Oncologic emergencies: diagnosis and treatment. Mayo Clin Proc. 2006 Jun;81(6): 835-48.*

#9

Which of the following factors is thought to be a high risk criteria in the patient with a neutropenic fever?

A. ANC ≥ 1000/mL

B. Absolute monocyte count ≥ 1000/mL

C. Hypotension

D. Duration of neutropenia > 8 days

E. Peak temperature < 39 °C

#9

Answer: C

Carefully selected patients with neutropenic fever may be treated in the outpatient setting. The MASCC score with the following criteria helps stratify patients.

1. Burden of febrile neutropenia with no or mild symptoms
2. No hypotension (systolic blood pressure > 90 mmHg)
3. No chronic obstructive pulmonary disease
4. Solid tumor or hematologic malignancy with no previous fungal infections
5. No dehydration requiring parenteral fluids
6. Burden of febrile neutropenia with moderate symptoms
7. Outpatient status at onset of fever
8. Age < 60 years

Close follow-up and unrestricted access to health care personnel are essential when patients are receiving outpatient therapy for neutropenic fever. A MASCC score ≥21 identifies low-risk patients with a positive predictive value of 91%, specificity of 68% and sensitivity of 71%.

- *Klastersky J, et al. The Multinational Association for Supportive Care in Cancer Risk Index: A Multinational Scoring System for Identifying Low-Risk Febrile Neutropenic Cancer Patients. J Clin Onc. 18: 3038-3051. full text*

- *Freifeld A, et al. Clinical Practice Guideline for the Use of Antimicrobial Agents in Neutropenic Patients with Cancer: 2010 Update by the Infectious Diseases Society of America. Clin Infect Dis. 2011 Feb 15; 52(4):e56-93. full text*

#10

Which of the following is a complication of massive transfusion?

A. Coagulopathy

B. Hypothermia

C. Acidosis

D. Electrolyte imbalances

E. Acute lung injury

F. All of the above

#10

Answer: F

Massive transfusion (MT) is associated with significant complications. The most commonly associated complications include acidosis, hypothermia, and coagulopathies. Patients may also develop hypocalcemia, hypomagnesemia, hypokalemia, hyperkalemia, citrate toxicity, and transfusion-associated acute lung injury. Once definitive control of hemorrhage has been established, a restrictive approach to blood transfusion should be implemented to minimize further complications and risk of infection.

- *Sihler KC, Napolitano LM. Complications of massive transfusion. Chest. 2010 Jan; 137(1): 209-20. full text*

#11

Massive transfusion protocols are being developed to optimize mortality and morbidity outcome in response to hemorrhagic shock. What is the optimal ratio of packed red blood cell: FFP: platelets when massive transfusion is warranted?

A. 1:1:1

B. 6:2:1

C. 4:1:1

D. 3:2:1

E. 2:1:1

#11

Answer: A

Massive transfusion protocols (MTP) in the civilian hospitals have changed to include plasma (fresh-frozen plasma [FFP]) and platelets as a result of current military recommendations to use component therapy at a 1:1:1 ratio of packed red blood cells to FFP to platelets.

Dente CJ, et al examined the results of implementation of a 1:1:1 ratio (RBC:FFP:platelets) when compared to a similar cohort prior to the 1:1:1 strategy. These patients were those requiring massive transfusions > 10 red blood cell (RBC) in the first 24 hours of hospitalization before instituting the new MTP. The patients in the new MTP received an average of 23.7 RBC and 15.6 FFP transfusions compared with 22.8 RBC ($p = 0.67$) and 7.6 FFP ($p < 0.001$) transfusions in pre-MTP patients. Early crystalloid usage dropped from 9.4 L (pre-MTP) to 6.9 L (MTP) ($p = 0.006$). Overall, patient mortality was markedly improved at 24 hours, from 36% in the pre-MTP group to 17% in the MTP group ($p = 0.008$) and at 30 days (34% mortality MTP group vs. 55% mortality in pre-MTP group, $p = 0.04$).

Blunt trauma survival improvements were more marked and more sustained than victims of penetrating trauma. Early deaths from coagulopathic bleeding occurred in 4 of 13 patients in the MTP group vs. 21 of 31 patients in the pre-MTP group ($p = 0.023$). Their conclusion was that aggressive use of FFP and platelets reduces 24-hour mortality and early coagulopathy in patients with trauma. Reduction in 30 day mortality was only seen after blunt trauma (not penetrating trauma) in this small subset.

The PROPPR trial also demonstrated that a 1:1:1 transfusion strategy did not result in significant differences in mortality at 24 hours or at 30 days. In post-hoc analysis there was a decrease in death by exsanguination in the first 24 hours in the 1:1:1 group.

- *Dente CJ, et al. Improvements in early mortality and coagulopathy are sustained better in patients with blunt trauma after institution of a massive transfusion protocol in a civilian level I trauma center. J Trauma. 2009 Jun; 66(6): 1616-24.*

- *Holcomb JB, et al. Transfusion of Plasma, Platelets, and Red Blood Cells in a 1:1:1 vs a 1:1:2 Ratio and Mortality in Patients With Severe Trauma The PROPPR Randomized Clinical Trial. JAMA. 2015; 313(5):471-482. full text*

- *Emcrit - The PROPPR trial with John Holcomb http://emcrit.org/podcasts/proppr/*

#12

Regarding infections in solid-organ transplant recipients, which of the following statements is FALSE?

A. It is more difficult to recognize infection in transplant recipients than in persons with normal immune function, since signs and symptoms of infection are often diminished.

B. There are no noninfectious causes of fever in transplant recipients.

C. Transplant patients are susceptible to a broad spectrum of potential pathogens, and infection often progresses rapidly.

D. A high sensitive CRP is an assay that can accurately measure a transplant patient's risk of infection.

E. Epidemiologic exposures can be divided into 4 overlapping categories: donor-derived infections, recipient-derived infections, nosocomial infections, and community infections.

#12

Answer: D

A, B, C, and E are true. The risk of infection after transplantation changes over time, particularly with modifications in immunosuppression. Unfortunately, no decision rules or lab values accurately measure a patient's risk of infection. The risk of missing an infection must be weighted with the risk of exposing a patient to an infection within the hospital. Consultation should occur with the patient's transplant physician.

- *Fishman JA. Infection in solid-organ transplant recipient. NEJM. 2007 Dec 20; 357(25): 2601-14. full text*

#13

Regarding infection in solid organ transplant recipients, which of the following statements are TRUE?

(Choose three answers.)

A. The routine evaluation of donors for infectious disease relies on antibody detection for common infections. Since the sensitivity of these tests are 100%, infections derived from donors no longer occurs.

B. Marijuana use is associated with infection with aspergillus.

C. Raising pigeons is associated with Cryptococcus neoformans infection.

D. Among transplant recipients, there is a 50 times increased rate of infection of Histoplasma and Tuberculosis.

E. Some patients who have HCV before liver transplantation are cured after the transplant and have no evidence of HCV.

#13

Answer: B, C, and D

Who knew? Marijuana use is associated with aspergillus infection in immunosupressed patients! Since seroconversion may not occur during acute infections and the sensitivity of these tests is not 100%, some active infections remain undetected. Some organs that contain unidentified pathogens will inevitably be implanted. The course of HCV infection after liver transplantation is discouraging, but with more effective antiviral therapies today, the outlook is good.

. *Fishman JA. Infection in solid-organ transplant recipient. NEJM. 2007 Dec 20; 357(25): 2601-14. full text*

#14

Regarding infection in solid organ transplant recipients, which of the following statements is TRUE regarding the use of trimethoprim-sulfamethoxazole?

A. Used for prophylaxis against pneumocystis pneumonia.

B. Used for prophylaxis against toxoplasma gondii

C. Used for prophylaxis against Isospora belli

D. Used for prophylaxis against Cyclospora cayetanensis, as well as for many nocardia and listeria species

E. All of the above

#14

Answer: E

Most transplant centers use trimethoprim-sulfamethoxazole prophylaxis for all of these pathogens. Low-doses are well tolerated and should be used unless there is evidence that the patient has an allergy or interstitial nephritis.

- *Fishman JA. Infection in solid-organ transplant recipient. NEJM. 2007 Dec 20; 357(25): 2601-14. full text*

#15

Regarding infection in solid organ transplant recipients, which of the following statements is TRUE?

A. CMV can cause invasive disease.

B. CMV can cause secondary immune phenomena.

C. CMV syndrome is characterized by fever, weakness, arthralgia, and myelosuppression.

D. Invasive disease usually occurs during the first year after completion of prophylaxis and is manifested most often as fever and neutropenia.

E. All of the above

#15

Answer: E

CMV may cause invasive disease and secondary immune complications. CMV syndrome is characterized by fever, weakness, myalgia, arthralgia, and myelosuppression. Infection with CMV can also cause end-organ disease, such as nephritis, hepatitis, carditis, colitis, pneumonitis, retinitis, and encephalitis.

- *Fishman JA. Infection in solid-organ transplant recipient. N Eng J Med. 2007 Dec 20;357(25): 2601-14. full text*

#16

Regarding infection in solid organ transplant recipients, which of the following statements is TRUE?

(Choose three answers.)

A. PTLD, or post-transplantation lymphoproliferative disorder, although serious, only has a mortality of < 1%.

B. Risk factors for PTLD include EBV infection after transplantation from seropositive donors.

C. Polyomaviruses, such as the JC virus has been associated with PML, but fortunately, there are effective antiviral therapies.

D. PTLD can be associated with intestinal obstruction.

E. Clinical presentations of PTLD associated with EBV can include unexplained fever, mono-like syndrome and GI bleeding.

#16

Answer: B, D, and E

Posttransplant lymphoproliferative disease occurs in 3-10% of adults who are solid-organ transplant recipients and carries a mortality rate of 40-60%. Complications from PTLD include:

1. Fever of unknown origin
2. Mononucleosis-like syndrome
3. Gastrointestinal bleeding
4. Intestinal obstruction, or perforation
5. Abdominal-mass lesions
6. Hepatitis and Pancreatitis
7. CNS disease

Polyomaviruses have been identified in transplant recipients in association with nephropathy (BK-associated nephropathy), and the JC virus is associated with progressive multifocal leukoencephalopathy. Unfortunately, no effective antiviral therapies exist for polyomaviruses.

- *Fishman JA. Infection in solid-organ transplant recipient. N Eng J Med. 2007 Dec 20; 357(25): 2601-14. full text*

INFECTIOUS DISEASE

#1

Which of the following statements about Dengue infection is FALSE?

A. There are four closely related but serologically distinct dengue viruses, called DEN-1, DEN-2, DEN-3, and DEN-4, of the genus Flavivirus.

B. Since there is only transient and weak cross-protection among the four serotypes, people living in an area of endemic dengue can be infected with all four, dengue serotypes during their lifetime.

C. The clinical manifestations of dengue range from asymptomatic infection, self-limited dengue fever, and dengue hemorrhagic fever with shock syndrome.

D. The risk of severe disease is much higher in primary dengue infection rather than sequential infection.

E. Symptoms typically develop between four and seven days after the bite of an infected mosquito, although the incubation period may range from 3 to 14 days.

#1

Answer: D

The risk of severe disease is much higher in recurrent rather than primary dengue infection. Classic dengue fever (DF) is an acute febrile illness with headache and musculoskeletal pain, often called "break-bone fever." Symptoms typically develop 4 - 7 days after the bite of an infected mosquito, but incubation can be as long as 2 weeks. Due to the consistent incubation period, the disease is unlikely in patients presenting with onset greater than 14 days after returning from a dengue-endemic country.

- *CDC Dengue http://www.cdc.gov/dengue/clinicalLab/index.html*

#2

Regarding the tuberculin PPD test, which of the following statements is FALSE?

(Choose two answers.)

A. A positive PPD may indicate exposure to tuberculosis.

B. If a PPD is positive, then it always indicates active disease.

C. If a PPD is negative, then it rules out active disease.

D. 5 units of PPD are injected intradermally during the PPD test.

E. Anergy may occur in HIV patients.

#2

Answer: B and C

Mantoux skin testing using purified protein derivative (PPD) is generally the first line of investigation for exposure to tuberculosis, with approximately 85% of patients with tuberculosis developing skin induration of >10 mm (a positive test). Typically, 5 units of PPD is injected into the skin with positivity based on the size of the wheal and patient specific criteria. The test is considered positive at:

- >5mm in HIV patients, or those who are immunosuppressed
- >10mm in patients at high risk for exposure such as foreign born, contact with family members who have tuberculosis, healthcare works or children < 4 years old
- >15mm in all other patients

Note that a positive Mantoux skin test indicates infection with M tuberculosis, but it does not indicate the activity of the infection.

- *Rosen's Emergency Medicine - Concepts and Clinical Practice. 8th edition. 2013. Chapter 134: Tick Borne Illness. 1816.*
- *CDC - Tuberculin Skin Testing http://www.cdc.gov/tb/publications/factsheets/testing/skintesting.htm*

#3

Regarding Rocky Mountain Spotted Fever (RMSF), which of the following statements is FALSE?

A. RMSF is limited to the Rocky Mountain area.

B. RMSF is an acute infectious disease caused by Rickettsia rickettsii and transmitted by the bites of several species of ticks (Dermacentor andersoni, Dermacentor variabilis, and Amblyomma).

C. The organisms can be introduced directly into the skin by a tick bite or may enter broken skin with the tick's feces.

D. RMSF is seen most commonly in the late spring and early summer.

E. The rash appears between the second and sixth days, beginning peripherally on the wrists, ankles, and forearms as a maculopapular rash extending to the torso, palms, and soles.

#3

Answer: A

RMSF is not limited to the Rocky Mountain area and occurs most commonly in the United States in the South Atlantic and Western, South-Central states. The disease is manifested clinically by fever, rash, myalgias, and headache. There is a broad spectrum of disease which range from mild to life threatening disease. RMSF is most commonly seen in the late spring and early summer. Note that the rash may be absent in 12 to 17% of the cases.

- *Rosen's Emergency Medicine - Concepts and Clinical Practice. 8th edition. 2013. Chapter 134: Tick Borne Illness. 1798-1802.*

#4

Which of the following statements about mammalian bites is FALSE?

A. Antibiotics are effective in preventing infection from bite wounds when used in certain clinical scenarios.

B. Prophylaxis is indicated in all human bites.

C. Prophylaxis is indicated in all cat and dog bite wounds.

D. Primary treatment for wounds involves careful assessment of function and control of blood loss.

E. It is important to determine the extent of the bite and any involvement to underlying tendons, neurovascular bundles, or joint spaces.

#4

Answer: C

According to a Cochrane review and meta-analysis on antibiotics in mammalian bites, the use of prophylactic antibiotics was associated with a statistically significant reduction in the rate of infection after bites by humans.

- Prophylactic antibiotics did not appear to reduce the rate of infection after bites by cats or dogs.
- Prophylactic antibiotics was associated with a statistically significant reduction in the rate of infection after bites by humans.
- Wound type (eg, laceration or puncture) did not appear to influence the effectiveness of the antibiotics.
- Prophylactic antibiotics were associated with a statistically significant reduction in the rate of infection in hand bites (odds ratio 0.10; 95% confidence interval [CI] 0.01 to 0.86); the number needed to treat was 4 (95% CI 2 to 50).

There is evidence that prophylactic antibiotics reduce the risk of infection **after human bites**, but not in cat or dog bites. **In bites to the hand**, there was a decrease in rates of infection (for all mammalian bites).

Pasteurella, Staphylococcus, Streptococcus, and Bacteroides are among the most common mammalian oral flora involved in infections after bites.

- *LLSA 2006: Turner TW. Do mammalian bites warrant antibiotic prophylaxis? Ann of Emerg Med. 2004 Sep ;44(3): 274-6. full text*

- *Medeiros I, Saconato H. Antibiotic prophylaxis for mammalian bites. Cochrane Database Syst Rev. 2001;(2):CD001738.*

#5

A healthy 35-year-old women presents with 3 days of diarrhea which is watery and non bloody. She has intermittent abdominal pain that is cramping in quality. Yesterday he had a fever of 38.7°C (101.7°F). Which of the following statements is FALSE regarding infectious diarrhea?

A. Regardless of the causative agent, initial therapy should always favor oral rehydration.

B. Whereas appropriate antibiotics are effective in the treatment of Shigellosis, Traveler's diarrhea, C. difficile and Campylobacter, antibiotics may prolong the duration of shedding of Salmonella.

C. Loperamide is the antimotility agent of choice for patients who present with inflammatory, bloody diarrhea.

D. The protozoal pathogens that are most frequently associated with diarrhea that persists for more than 7 to 10 days, both in the United States and worldwide, are Giardia and Cryptosporidium.

E. In immunocompetent patients with Campylobacter, erythromycin can decrease the duration of illness if given within four days.

#5

Answer: C

Loperamide is an antimotility agent that inhibits intestinal peristalsis and has antisecretory properties, but does not have opioid-like properties like other antimotility agents such as diphenoxylate and codeine. It will reduce the duration of diarrhea, but in patients with invasive inflammatory causes of diarrhea such as Shigella, it may increase the risk of hemolytic uremic syndrome and prolong the period of bacterial infection. In patients with C. difficile, it can also increase the risk of toxic megacolon.

History and physical should guide management in the majority of patients with diarrheal symptoms. For example, recent antibiotic use or hospitalization suggests C. difficile. C. difficile, however, has also been reported in patients without any history of antibiotic exposure. The presence of bloody diarrhea should warrant further testing for Shigella, Salmonella, and Campylobacter.

- Salmonella should be suspected in patients with sickle cell disease.
- Recent travel increases the risk for Enterotoxigenic *Escherichia coli* (ETEC) and may warrant a single dose of a quinolone antibiotic if severely symptomatic.
- Travelers to southern Asia are at risk for quinolone-resistant Campylobacter, in addition to ETEC.
- Empiric treatment for inflammatory diarrhea can be considered, based on exposure history to Salmonella, Shigella or Campylobacter infection.

- *LLSA 2006: Thielman NM, et al. Acute Infectious Diarrhea. N Eng J Med. 2004 Jan 1; 350(1): 38-47. full text*
- *CDC Travelers Diarrhea http://www.cdc.gov/ncidod/dbmd/diseaseinfo/travelersdiarrhea_g.htm*

#6

You are seeing an immigrant from India who presents with bilateral cervical adenopathy. Approximately what percentage of patients present with extrapulmonary tuberculosis of the head and neck?

A. 50%

B. 40%

C. 15%

D. 10%

#6

Answer: C

Approximately 1.5% of new tuberculosis worldwide manifests as extrapulmonary TB, and 15% of those cases occur in the head and neck. Patients with TB lymphadenitis have enlarged bilateral cervical nodes that are painful and warm, and often affect the posterior cervical chain.

- *Rosen's Emergency Medicine - Concepts and Clinical Practice. 8th edition. 2013. Chapter 135: Tuberculosis. 1818 - 1821.*

#7

The benefits of dexamethasone treatment for moderate-to-severe croup are well established. Most children with croup have mild symptoms. Which of the following statements is FALSE?

A. At least 60% of children with croup who present for emergency care have mild symptoms and are routinely discharged without observation or treatment.

B. Corticosteroids are effective in moderate-to-severe croup, resulting in reductions in the frequency and duration of intubation and hospitalization.

C. The risk of corticosteroid administration outweighs the benefit for patients with MILD croup and should be avoided.

D. Corticosteroid treatment for lung disease in premature neonates has been associated with long-term adverse effects on growth and neuromotor and cognitive function.

E. Repeated short courses of oral corticosteroids in children with asthma are not associated with long-term negative effects on bone metabolism, bone density, or adrenal function.

#7

Answer: C

Bjornsen C, et al. conducted a double-blind trial at four pediatric emergency departments, which randomly assigned children with mild croup to receive either dexamethasone (0.6 mg/kg) or placebo. The children with mild croup were defined by a score of 2 on the Westley croup scoring system. The primary outcome was return to a medical care provider for croup within seven days after treatment, and secondary outcomes were croup symptoms on days 1, 2, and 3 after treatment.

Bouncebacks were significantly lower in the dexamethasone group (7.3% vs. 15.3%, $p<0.001$), and there were also decreased time to symptoms resolution ($p=0.003$), less lost sleep ($p<0.001$), and decreased parental stress ($p<0.001$).

The authors concluded that for children with mild croup, dexamethasone is an effective treatment that results in consistent and small but important clinical and economic benefits. Therefore the current recommendations are for a single dose of dexamethasone as initial treatment of croup.

- *LLSA 2006: Bjornsen CL, et al. A randomized trial of a single dose of oral dexamethasone for mild croup. N Eng J Med. 2004 Sep 23;351(13):1306-13. full text*

#8

When comparing infection rates between using clean nonsterile gloves and sterile gloves in the repair of uncomplicated traumatic lacerations, using clean non-sterile gloves is associated with an infection rate that is:

A. Statistically significantly higher than the rate when sterile gloves were used

B. Significantly lower than the rate when sterile gloves were used

C. Not different in a clinically important way

#8

Answer: C

Perelman, et al. in a prospective multicenter trial enrolled 816 individuals who were randomized to have their wounds repaired, using sterile or clean nonsterile gloves. At the time of suture removal, wounds were evaluated for the presence or absence of infection. Follow-up was obtained for 98% of the sterile gloves group and 96.6% of the clean gloves group. There was no statistically significant difference in the incidence of infection between the 2 groups. The infection rate in the sterile gloves group was 6.1% (95% confidence interval [CI] 3.8% to 8.4%) and was 4.4% in the clean gloves group (95% CI 2.4% to 6.4%). The relative risk of infection was 1.37 (95% CI 0.75 to 2.52). This study demonstrated that there is no clinically important difference in infection rates between using clean nonsterile gloves and sterile gloves during the repair of uncomplicated traumatic lacerations. There may also be an additional time and cost savings for using nonsterile gloves.

- *LLSA 2006: Perelman VS, et al. Sterile versus nonsterile gloves for repair of uncomplicated lacerations in the emergency department: a randomized controlled trial. Ann Emerg Med. 2004 Mar; 43(3): 362-70.*

#9

You are treating a patient with a small cutaneous abscess on his arm. Which of the following is the most appropriate management strategy?

A. Simply perform an incision and drainage.

B. Perform an incision and drainage and start broad-spectrum antibiotics.

C. Perform an incision and drainage and start antibiotics specifically targeted for MRSA.

D. Recommend warm soaks and arm elevation.

E. None of the above

#9

Answer: A

A review of the literature found 5 studies and 1 abstract spanning over a 30-year period, which address the issue of clinical outcomes of abscess incision and drainage with or without outpatient oral antibiotics. The studies concluded that patients treated with I & D alone have infection resolution at the same rate as those with I & D plus antibiotics. The only caveat is in patients with significant cellulitis associated with the abscess. None of the studies addressed abscesses with an associated cellulitis so no firm conclusion can be extrapolated in that situation.

Also, immunocompromised patients were not included in one study, and abscesses were not clearly defined, placing some limitations on the data. Still, in patients with simple cutaneous abscesses, despite the prevalence of methicillin-resistant staphylococcus aureus, I & D without antibiotics is appropriate and effective.

- *LLSA 2009: Hankin A, Everett WW. Are Antibiotics Necessary After Incision and Drainage of a Cutaneous Abscess? Annals of Emerg Med.2007 Jul; 50(1): 49-51.*

#10

The risk factor most predictive of Methicillin Resistant Staph Aureus (MRSA) infection is:

A. Presence of a furunculosis

B. Age

C. Injection drug use history

D. Hospitalization history

E. HIV status

#10

Answer: A

Frazee B, et al. conducted a prospective observational study involving a convenience sample of patients who presented with skin and soft tissue infections to a single urban public hospital ED in California. Cultures were obtained from the nares and the infection site to determine if the wound and patient were infected and colonized by MRSA.

- White race and furuncle (superficial abscess) were associated with both MRSA colonization and infection.
- Factors not associated with MRSA were age, income, incarceration history, hospitalization history, injection drug use status and frequency, injection drug use hygiene habits, known MRSA contact, antibiotic use history, skin disease history, and HIV status.
- Homelessness and a recent history of multiple abscesses were associated only with colonization and not with MRSA infection.

Although the ability to predict if a patient has MRSA is difficult, patients with superficial abscesses are more likely to have MRSA than those with a cellulitis.

- *LLSA 2007: Frazee BW, et al. High prevalence of methicillin resistant staph aureus in emergency department skin and soft tissue infections. Ann Emerg Med. 2005 Mar; 45(3): 311-20. full text*

#11

A 75 year old female who underwent a pacemaker insertion 8 days ago presents with fevers and pain over the insertion site. The site looks erythematous, warm, and tender. All of the following are appropriate management steps, EXCEPT:

A. Start the patient on oral cefalexin and sulfamethoxazole/trimethoprim and have her return for a wound check in 3 days.

B. Update her tetanus vaccination status, if she is not up to date.

C. Administer a dose of parenteral antibiotics to cover for staph aureus both (MSSA and MRSA) while the patient is in the emergency department.

D. Consult the surgeon or interventional cardiologist who placed the pacemaker for possible removal and replacement.

E. Consider obtaining an ultrasound to look for an abscess.

#11

Answer: A

Infections of pacemakers occur in approximately 6 to 15% of patients, with staph species being the most common pathogens. In the patient presenting with fever and redness and tenderness over the pulse generator pocket, the diagnosis is pacemaker infection until proven otherwise. Pacemaker site infection requires IV antibiotics and evaluation for device removal.

- *Rosen's Emergency Medicine - Concepts and Clinical Practice. 8th edition. 2013. Chapter 80: Implantable Cardiac Devices. 1067.*

#12

An 11 year old boy who had been hiking in the Rocky Mountains for vacation is brought in by his parents for fevers, myalgias, headache, and a single painless target lesion. You suspect Colorado Tick Fever (CTF). Which of the following statements about CTF is FALSE?

A. The pathogen of CTF is a double-stranded RNA arbovirus of the Reoviridae family.

B. Leukocytosis will be present on the CBC.

C. The virus is spread by the Rocky Mountain wood tick (Dermacentor andersoni), although blood transfusion related infection has also been reported.

D. CTF is benign and self-limiting.

#12

Answer: B

CTF virus infects hematopoietic cells, causing a leukopenia. The hallmark of CTF is a leukocyte count less than 4000 with neutropenia more pronounced than lymphopenia. Thrombocytopenia is occasionally seen, as well. All of the other statements are true.

- *Rosen's Emergency Medicine - Concepts and Clinical Practice. 8th edition. 2013. Chapter 134: Tick Borne Illness. 1806 -1807.*

#13

Erysipelas is characterized by all of the following EXCEPT:

A. Caused almost exclusively by group A streptococci, although occasional cases are due to Staph aureus

B. Most commonly occurs in infants and young children

C. Diffuse blanching across skin surfaces and poorly defined margins

D. In adults, it is likely to occur in the setting of venous stasis, lymphedema, diabetes, or alcohol abuse.

E. Untreated lesions can form bullae that break down and leave raw, weeping surfaces.

#13

Answer: C

In contrast to common cellulitis, the lesion of erysipelas is sharply demarcated, indurated, easily palpable, and has a raised border. Characteristically, it is also shiny red. All of the other statements are true.

- *Rosen's Emergency Medicine - Concepts and Clinical Practice. 8th edition. 2013. Chapter 120: Dermatologic Presentations. 1566.*

#14

You suspect that your patient has herpetic whitlow. True statements about this entity include all of the following EXCEPT:

(Choose two answers.)

A. Topical acyclovir has been shown to be effective.

B. Incision and drainage should be performed as soon as possible.

C. It is a viral infection of the fingertip caused by type 1 and type 2 herpes simplex viruses.

D. The infection most often affects the distal pulp space and occasionally the proximal and lateral nail folds.

E. The distal pulp space usually remains soft, and this helps to differentiate it from a felon, in which there is tense swelling of the distal pulp space.

#14

Answer: A and B

Herpetic whitlow is a self resolving herpes simplex infection of the distal finger. It can easily be mistaken for a paronychia or a digital infection. It should not involve the pulp space, and careful history and presence of a healing or new vesicle can aid in distinguishing it from a bacterial infection. Incision and drainage should not be performed. Simple wound dressing and daily cleaning is sufficient to prevent secondary bacterial infection. The use of oral acyclovir, famciclovir, or valacyclovir has been reported to be effective in recurrent attacks.

- *Rosen's Emergency Medicine - Concepts and Clinical Practice. 8th edition. 2013. Chapter 50: Hand. 566.*

#15

Which of the following is NOT part of the official criteria for the systemic inflammatory response syndrome (SIRS)?

A. Temperature > 38.5°C or < 35°C

B. HR > 100 bpm

C. RR > 20/min or $PCO_2 < 32$ mm Hg

D. WBC > 12,000 cell/mm^3 or < 4,000 cell/mm^3

E. 10% bandemia

#15

Answer: B

SIRS is clinically recognized by the presence of two or more of the above criteria, except for the HR cutoff. HR > 90 bpm meets the criteria.

- *Rosen's Emergency Medicine - Concepts and Clinical Practice. 8th edition. 2013. Chapter 138: Sepsis Syndromes. 1864.*

#16

Sepsis is defined as SIRS in response to a documented infection (culture or gram stain of blood, sputum, urine, or normally sterile body fluid), or which of the following:

A. Wound with purulent discharge

B. Obvious pneumonia on chest X-ray

C. Intra-abdominal bowel contents found during surgery

D. All of the above

#16

Answer: E

Sepsis is defined as SIRS in response to a documented infection (culture positive) or infection identified by visual inspection.

- *Rosen's Emergency Medicine - Concepts and Clinical Practice. 8th edition. 2013. Chapter 138: Sepsis Syndromes. 1864.*

#17

Dengue hemorrhagic fever (DHF) is the most serious manifestation of dengue virus infection and can be associated with shock. The four cardinal features of DHF include all of the following features, EXCEPT:

A. Increased vascular permeability

B. Fever

C. Headache

D. Hemorrhage

E. Marked thrombocytopenia (less than 100,000/ mm^3)

#17

Answer: C

Dengue hemorrhagic fever (DHF) is the most serious manifestation of dengue virus infection and can be associated with circulatory failure and shock.

Cardinal features of DHF, as defined by the World Health Organization (WHO), include:

1. Fever lasting 2 to 7 days
2. Marked thrombocytopenia (less than 100,000 cells/mm3)
3. Increased vascular permeability (plasma leakage syndrome)
4. Any hemorrhage

The term dengue shock syndrome (DSS) is used when shock is present along with these four criteria.

- *Rosen's Emergency Medicine - Concepts and Clinical Practice. 8th edition. 2013. Chapter 130: Viral Illnesses Sepsis Syndromes. 1738 - 1741.*
- *CDC Dengue and Hemorrhagic Fever http://1.usa.gov/14tkqZg*

#18

All of the following statements are true about malaria, EXCEPT:

A. Human malaria is caused by four species of Plasmodium: P. falciparum, P. vivax, P. ovale, and P. malariae.

B. Humans are the only important malarial reservoir, and there are no free-living plasmodia.

C. Malaria transmission is predominantly via the bite of a female Anopheles sp. mosquito, which occurs mainly between dusk and dawn.

D. P. falciparum infects only young red blood cells (reticulocytes), thereby limiting parasitemia levels to one to two percent.

E. The gold standard for the diagnosis of malaria is the combination of thick and thin blood smears examined via light microscopy.

#18

Answer: D

P. falciparum can invade red cells of all ages, causing high levels of parasitemia affecting as great as 50% of red blood cells (RBCs). P. vivax and P. ovale only affect reticulocytes and cause less parasitemia. Patient at greatest risk from the parasitemia are the elderly, immunocompromised, asplenic, children, pregnant women, and those with significant comorbidities. Diagnosis is based on thick and thin blood smears. Thick smears are the most sensitive, while the thin smear allows morphologic species determinations. The first smears are positive in 95% of cases, but smears should be repeated every 6 to 12 hours to exclude the diagnosis.

- *Rosen's Emergency Medicine - Concepts and Clinical Practice. 8th edition. 2013. Chapter 133: Parasitic Infections. 1769-1776.*

#19

Regarding traveler's diarrhea (TD), which of the following statements is FALSE?

A. The mainstay of therapy for travelers' diarrhea is fluid replacement.

B. Travelers' diarrhea is the most common illness in persons traveling from resource-rich to resource-poor regions of the world.

C. More than 90% of illnesses in most geographic areas are caused by viruses.

D. Antimotility agents are usually not necessary for mild to moderate diarrhea and should not be used in severe diarrhea except in association with antibiotic therapy.

E. Episodes of travelers' diarrhea (TD) are nearly always benign and self-limited, but the dehydration that can complicate an episode may be severe and pose a greater health hazard than the illness itself.

#19

Answer: C

More than 90% of travelers diarrhea is caused by Enterotoxigenic Escherichia coli (ETEC). Other potential infectious bacteria are Salmonella spp., Campylobacter jejuni, and Shigella. Viruses compose a small percentage, with Rotaviruses being the most common. Traveler's diarrhea does not generally last more than five days. For non-complicated travelers diarrhea, routine stool cultures are not necessary. If patients have fever, bloody diarrhea and evidence of systemic illness, then stool cultures should be sent. Stool cultures should also be considered in immunocompromised patients or those with chronic symptoms. Antimicrobial therapy with a fluoroquinolone may shorten the disease duration, and antimotility agents may limit symptoms but can increase bacterial retention in patients with invasive diarrhea. The 2006 guidelines on travel medicine from the Infectious Diseases Society of America recommends the following oral agents as options for the treatment of travelers' diarrhea: norfloxacin, ciprofloxacin, ofloxacin, levofloxacin, azithromycin, or rifaximin – all for three days.

- *Hill D, et al. The practice of travel medicine: guidelines by the Infectious Diseases Society of America. Clin Infect Dis. 2006; 43(12): 1499-539. full text*

#20

Which of the follow statements are NOT consistent with your evaluation/management of a patient who sustained a human bite of the hand (fight bite) from a clenched-fist or closed-fist injury?

A. Any patient with a laceration or puncture in the vicinity of the MCP joint should have hand radiographs looking for fractures, dislocations, retained teeth and air in the joint.

B. The wound should be assessed and examined through the full range of motion.

C. Human bites should be irrigated and debrided.

D. If presenting within 4-8 hours of injury, human bites can be safely closed as long as you irrigate copiously.

E. Prophylactic antibiotics are recommended for coverage of polymicrobial infection including gram positive organisms and Eikenella.

#20

Answer: D

Infectious complications in human bites to the hand are reported in 25-50% of cases. Although there are no controlled studies on suturing human bites, the high rate of infection and complications suggest that the wound be left open. Healthy patients who present within 24 hours of injury without infection or tendon/bone/joint injury can be treated as an outpatient with close follow-up within 24 to 48 hours. High risk patients, delayed presentation, or deep structure involvement warrants prophylactic IV antibiotics and close observation.

- *Rosen's Emergency Medicine - Concepts and Clinical Practice. 8th edition. 2013. Chapter 50: Hand. 562.*

#21

A local farm-hand complains of fever, chills and myalgias. He states that he works on a dairy farm where there are sheep, goats and cows. You, of course consider Q Fever in your differential. Which of the following statements is NOT consistent with Q fever?

A. It is a tick-borne illness, (like other tick-borne illnesses, such as Lyme Disease, Tularemia and Rocky Mountain Spotted Fever), which occurs most commonly after a bite from an arthropod vector.

B. Clinical manifestations include severe retrobulbar headache, fever to 40 ºC or higher, chills, malaise, myalgias and chest pain.

C. Regarded primarily as a respiratory disease, it may cause chronic infection in the form of hepatitis and endocarditis.

D. As with other rickettsial diseases, tetracyclines and chloramphenicol are effective in treatment of acute Q Fever.

E. It is extremely infectious with a single inhaled organism sufficient to initiate infection and is considered a potential biological warfare agent.

#21

Answer: A

Q fever (Coxiella burnetii) are extremely resistant and can survive for long periods of time in inanimate environments. Diagnosis should be considered in a patient with a severe febrile illness without obvious cause, especially in someone with recent contact with sheep, cattle, goats or animal by products. Q fever was originally thought to be a rickettsial disease until it was discovered to be Coxiella. Unlike other rickettsial diseases, humans are most commonly infected by inhalation of aerosolized particles from contaminated environments. It is extremely infectious with a single inhaled organism sufficient to initiate infection. Thus, it has been considered a potential biological warfare agent. Most acute Q fever infections resolve without treatment; however, given the risk of chronic infection, treatment is advisable.

- *Rosen's Emergency Medicine - Concepts and Clinical Practice. 8th edition. 2013. Chapter 134: Tick Borne Illness. 1803-1804.*
- *CDC - Q Fever in Slaughterhouses http://www.cdc.gov/mmwr/preview/mmwrhtml/00000714.htm*

#22

Which of the following antibiotic agents used to treat skin and soft tissue infections (SSTI) is associated with inducible resistance?

A. Clindamycin

B. Linezolid

C. Minocycline

D. Vancomycin

#22

Answer: A

Clindamycin is an important adjunct to therapy for SSTI because of its ability to suppress bacterial toxin production, including streptococcal pyrogenic exotoxin A, Panton Valentine leukocidin (PVL), and staphylococcus enterotoxin B. However, MRSA may become resistant to clindamycin upon exposure to this drug via an inducible gene found in certain strains. The microbiology laboratory usually performs a disk diffusion test, known as a D-test to determine if inducible resistance is present.

- *Prabhu K, Rao S, Venkatakrishna R. Inducible clindamycin resistance in Staphylococcus aureus isolated from clinical samples. J Lab Physicians. 2011; 3(1): 25–27.*

#23

You are seeing a patient with a history of HIV who was started on HAART therapy 6 weeks ago and has signs of hepatosplenomegaly, pneumonitis, lymphadenitis, and an elevated calcium level. She was recently diagnosed with M. Avium complex. What is the most likely cause of this patient's presentation with MAC, hepatosplenomegaly, pneumonitis, lymphadenitis, and hypercalcemia?

A. HIV pneumonitis

B. PCP pneumonia

C. CNS lymphoma

D. Cryptococcal hepatitis

E. Immune Reconstitution Inflammatory Syndrome

#23

Answer: E

Immune reconstitution inflammatory syndrome (IRIS) represents a unique consequence of the initiation of HAART. The reconstitution of the immune system response by HAART can exacerbate otherwise dormant opportunistic pathogens or aggravate the symptoms of clinically apparent opportunistic disease. M. avium complex is the most likely disease to occur during IRIS and manifests with lymphadenitis, pneumonitis, hepatosplenomegaly, and hypercalcemia. However, any opportunistic infection can occur during reconstitution.

Risk factors associated with immune reconstitution inflammatory syndrome include:

1. Initial HAART therapy
2. Prior opportunistic infections
3. Rapid decrease in HIV viral load.

If IRIS occurs, it is more likely during the first 8 weeks of initiating HAART therapy. Treatment is aggressive supportive care with NSAIDS and occasionally steroids. HAART should not be routinely discontinued.

- *Venkat A, et al. Care of the HIV-positive patient in the emergency department in the era of highly active antiretroviral therapy. Ann Emerg Med. 2008 Sep; 52(3): 274-85. full text*

#24

Which of the following is the most common cause of erysipelas?

A. Enterococcus faecalis

B. Staphylococcus aureus

C. Staphylococcus epidermidis

D. Streptococcus pyogenes

#24

Answer: D

Strep pyogenes is the most common cause of erysipelas, and this infection is characterized by acute onset of skin erythema associated with fever and lymphangitis. The classic skin lesion is raised with well-demarcated borders. It is caused by prominent lymphatic compromise of the affected area. Erysipelas most often develops on the lower extremities, contrary to past trends when facial involvement was the most common presentation. Colonization of the skin, dermatophyte infection between the toes or of the toenails, chronic venous stasis and preexisting leg ulcers are all predisposing factors for developing erysipelas. Because of the superficial nature of the disease, subsequent bacteremia is rarely found, making blood culture collection unnecessary in most cases.

- *Rosen's Emergency Medicine - Concepts and Clinical Practice. 8th edition. 2013. Chapter 137: Skin and Soft Tissue Infections. 1852.*

#25

A patient with known HIV and CD4 count of 195 presents with diarrhea for the last 3 days that has been profuse. He does not have any vomiting, fever, or abdominal pain. He has been taking his HAART medications and denies any recent travel. On examination, the patient appears to be dehydrated with dry mucus membranes and tachycardia. The most likely etiology of his diarrhea is:

A. Clostridium difficile

B. Candida

C. Mycobacterium

D. Cryptosporidium

E. Microsporidia

#25

Answer: A

Gastrointestinal ailments remain among the most common complaints in HIV-infected patients. HAART has resulted in a decrease in incidence of C. albicans esophagitis, with a resultant decrease in the use of antifungal medications by HIV-infected patients. In a patient on HAART therapy, Clostridium difficile has become the most likely bacterial pathogen. Up to 36% of HIV-infected patients with acute diarrhea requiring hospitalization likely have C. difficile.

Emergency Department treatment should focus on volume resuscitation, and appropriate stool studies should be sent. In patients with advanced AIDS who are at risk for Cryptosporidium parvum and Microsporidia species, special stool studies are required for diagnosis (acid-fast stain for Cryptosporidium parvum, light microscopy for Microsporidia species).

- *Venkat A, et al. Care of the HIV patient in the era of highly active antiretroviral treatment. Ann Emerg Med. 2008 Sep; 52(3): 274-85. full text*

#26

All of the following statements are true regarding the H1N1 virus, EXCEPT:

A. It is spread via large particle aerosol and direct contact with surfaces contaminated with droplets contaminated with H1N1.

B. It was considered a pandemic by the WHO.

C. Patients are considered contagious from one day prior to onset of symptoms to 2 days after symptom onset.

D. Typical clinical manifestations include fever, cough, sore throat, headache, myalgias, and gastrointestinal symptoms.

#26

Answer: C

In 2009, an outbreak of H1N1 influenza A virus infection was detected in Mexico, followed by outbreaks in other countries. On June 11, 2009, the World Health Organization raised its pandemic alert level to the highest level, phase 6, indicating widespread community transmission on at least two continents. Influenza virus is transmitted via large-particle aerosols, as well as by contact with surfaces that have been contaminated with respiratory droplets. Patients with H1N1 influenza A virus infection are contagious from one day prior to the development of signs and symptoms until resolution of fever. The patient is contagious for 7 days after illness onset. During the 2009 pandemic, rapidly progressing pneumonia, respiratory failure, and acute respiratory distress syndrome were reported, in addition to the usual fever, cough, headache and myalgias.

- *CDC - 2009 H1N1 Flu. http://www.cdc.gov/h1n1flu/*
- *CDC. Outbreak of swine origin influenza A (H1N1) virus infection - Mexico, March-April 2009. MMWR. 2009; 58: 467–70. http://www.cdc.gov/mmwr/preview/mmwrhtml/mm58d0430a2.htm*

#27

Regarding diagnostic testing for the H1N1 virus, all of the following are true EXCEPT:

A. The rapid point-of-care test has a high sensitivity, and when a negative test is found, it is definitively negative.

B. In the United States, the recommended test to confirm the diagnosis of pandemic H1N1 influenza A virus is real-time reverse transcriptase (RT)-PCR for influenza A, B, H1, and H3.

C. The strain of H1N1 influenza A virus associated with the 2009 pandemic tests positive for influenza A and negative for H1 and H3 by real-time RT-PCR.

D. Isolation of pandemic H1N1 influenza A virus using culture is diagnostic, but culture is usually too slow to help guide clinical management.

E. A negative viral culture does not exclude pandemic H1N1 influenza A infection.

#27

Answer: A

In the United States, the recommended test to confirm the diagnosis of pandemic H1N1 influenza A virus is real-time reverse transcriptase (RT)-PCR for influenza A, B, H1, and H3. In general, RT-PCR is performed only when the results will substantially impact clinical management or when there is a recognized public health benefit. Isolation of pandemic H1N1 influenza A virus using culture is diagnostic, but culture is usually too slow to help guide clinical management. A negative viral culture does not exclude pandemic H1N1 influenza A infection. The sensitivity and specificity of rapid antigen testing for pandemic H1N1 influenza A virus infection have not been definitively established, but poor sensitivity has already been demonstrated for seasonal influenza. Based on limited data, the sensitivity of rapid antigen testing for detecting pandemic H1N1 influenza is approximately 50-70%. There are many false negative tests.

- *CDC 2009 H1N1 Flu. http://www.cdc.gov/h1n1flu/*
- *CDC Influenza and Laboratory Diagnostics http://www.cdc.gov/flu/professionals/diagnosis/labrolesprocedures.htm*

#28

Regarding treatment for H1N1, all of the following are true EXCEPT:

A. If the H1N1 strain is thought to be resistant to oseltamivir, then amantadine or rimantadine would be the recommended primary alternatives.

B. Ideally, the medication should be administered within 48 hours of symptom onset.

C. The CDC recommends treatment for all hospitalized patients with presumptive influenza and all patients who are at high risk for complications.

D. Among those children the greatest complication risk is in those < 2 years of age.

E. The treatment duration is 5 days.

#28

Answer: A

Antiviral therapy (with zanamivir or oseltamivir) is recommended by the CDC for all hospitalized patients with confirmed, probable, or suspected pandemic H1N1 influenza A virus infection and for patients at increased risk for complications. During the 2009 pandemic, patients with mild illness did not require testing or treatment unless they had risk factors for complications. The vast majority of strains of pandemic H1N1 influenza A virus circulating in 2009 were sensitive to the neuraminidase inhibitors (oseltamivir or zanamivir) but were resistant to amantadine and rimantadine. Thus, in locations where oseltamivir-resistant seasonal H1N1 influenza A virus is circulating, zanamivir is the preferred antiviral. Patients who are unable to take zanamivir in such a setting can be given the combination of an adamantane (rimantadine or amantadine) with oseltamivir. In addition to patients with underlying illnesses, all children younger than 5 years of age, particularly those less than 2 years of age, are at increased risk for complications of influenza.

- *CDC 2009 H1N1 Flu. http://www.cdc.gov/h1n1flu/*

#29

Since the advent of HAART, the incidence of oral candidiasis and CMV retinitis has:

A. Increased

B. Decreased

C. Stayed the same

D. Become epidemic

#29

Answer: B

Before the advent of HAART, esophageal candidiasis and cytomegalovirus retinitis were the most common manifestations of underlying HIV/AIDS. HAART has resulted in a decreased incidence of both conditions, with candidiasis reduced by up to 50% in population-based observational studies and Cytomegalovirus retinitis by up to 80%. Patients on HAART are generally no longer being prescribed prophylactic medication for candidiasis or Cytomegalovirus. However, patients receiving HAART are at increased risk of oral warts and continue to be at risk of HIV-related periodontal disease.

Immune reconstitution inflammatory syndrome from initiation of HAART places patients at risk for immune reconstitution vitritis and uveitis. Presentation can include vision loss and macular edema on on slit-lamp exam. Treatment involves corticosteroids and ophthalmology consult. Most patients have full visual recovery.

- *Venkat A, et al. Care of the HIV-positive patient in the emergency department in the era of highly active antiretroviral therapy. Ann Emerg Med. 2008 Sep; 52(3): 274-85. full text*

#30

HAART has changed the predominant neurologic disease manifestations in the HIV infected patient. Which of the following neurologic diseases has not decreased, however, since HAART was instituted?

A. Toxoplasma

B. Lymphoma

C. Cryptococcus

D. Progressive multifocal leukoencephalopathy

E. All of the above have decreased

#30

Answer: E

All the the nervous system infections associated with HIV/AIDS have decreased since widespread use of HAART. Prior to HAART therapy, opportunistic CNS infections (Toxoplasma gondii and C. neoformans) were the primary cause of neurologic disease in HIV patients. Progressive multifocal leukoencephalopathy caused by JC polyoma virus has also decreased, but still remains a cause of encephalitis in HIV/AIDS patients.

Patients with progressive multifocal leukoencephalopathy (PML) present with altered mental status, speech disturbances, visual deficits, gait difficulty, weakness, hemiparesis, and limb incoordination. Diagnosis can be suggestive on MRI but confirmed by CSF PCR. If a patient develops PML during immune reconstitution inflammatory syndrome, the MRI will reveal contrast-enhancing lesions, raising the concern for other entities such as CNS lymphoma and toxoplasmosis.

- *Venkat A, et al. Care of the HIV-positive patient in the emergency department in the era of highly active antiretroviral therapy. Ann Emerg Med. 2008 Sep; 52(3): 274-85. full text*

#31

Protease inhibitor use in HIV patients has been associated with:

A. Hyperlipidemia

B. Hyperglycemia

C. Truncal obesity

D. Atherosclerosis

E. All of the above

#31

Answer: E

All medications in the protease inhibitor class may cause hyperlipidemia, hyperglycemia, and truncal obesity. These effects may be contributing to the increasing cardiovascular disease and diabetes in aging HIV patients on long term HAART. Within the class of protease inhibitors, Ritonavir has the greatest association with these complications and Atazanavir the least. Protease inhibitor use is associated with an increased risk of atherogenic lipoprotein dysfunction and resultant atherosclerosis as well. There is a relative increased risk of 1.75 (95% CI 1.51 to 2.02) for acute myocardial infarction in HIV-infected patients and a 1.16 relative increased risk of MI of per year of protease inhibitor use (95% CI 1.10 to 1.23).

In evaluating patients for acute coronary syndrome, maintain an increased suspicion in younger patients who are on HAART, especially those who are on protease inhibitors.

- *Venkat A, et al. Care of the HIV-positive patient in the emergency department in the era of highly active antiretroviral therapy. Ann Emerg Med. 2008 Sep; 52(3): 274-85. full text*

#32

In a retrospective cohort study of HIV patients in the HAART era, which of the following two variables were associated with increased ED utilization?

(Choose two answers.)

A. Viral load

B. Income level

C. Age

D. Race

E. Gender

#32

Answer: A and B

In a retrospective cohort study of 356 HIV-positive adults, income level and mean viral load had a significant association ($p < 0.05$) with ED utilization. Of 155 ICD-9 ED discharge diagnoses, ill-defined symptoms/signs (25.2%), injury (18.7%), and musculoskeletal disorders (11.6%) were most prevalent. Of 450 ICD-9 hospital discharge diagnoses, endocrine/metabolic (13.3%), psychiatric (12.2%), infectious/parasitic (12%), and circulatory disorders (11.8%) were most prevalent.

- *Venkat A, et al. Care of the HIV-positive patient in the emergency department in the era of highly active antiretroviral therapy. Ann Emerg Med. 2008 Sep; 52(3): 274-85. full text*

#33

Regarding influenza, which of the following statements is TRUE?

(Choose two answers.)

A. It is diagnosed every month of the year somewhere in the world.

B. Myocarditis is a common complication of influenza.

C. Amantadine and rimantadine are effective against either type A or type B influenza.

D. If a neuraminidase inhibitor, such as oseltamivir (tamiflu) is used, the duration of clinical symptoms is shortened by 3 days.

E. In times of epidemic infection, the high prevalence of disease combined with the greater likelihood of false-negative test results may make empiric treatment based on clinical presentation alone a reasonable consideration in certain patient populations.

#33

Answer: A and E

Influenza is present at all times in various parts of the world depending on the season. In northern hemispheres, the flu season occurs from November through March. Tropical regions have reports of the virus active year-round. The most common complications are acute bronchitis, otitis media and secondary bacterial pneumonia, and acute dehydration. Rare complications include pericarditis, transverse myelitis, and Guillain-Barre syndrome.

Antiviral therapy include M2 protein inhibitors (amantadine and rimantadine) for influenza A virus, and neuraminidase inhibitors for both A and B types. Uses of these medications is controversial due to poor disclosure of all data from the pharmaceutical manufacturer, but studies show that the maximal clinical symptom duration is shortened by about 1 day.

In one prospective study of adults presenting with an influenza-like-illness when the prevalence of influenza was high, rapid testing was NO better than clinical judgment alone in making the diagnosis of influenza. During peak influenza activity, a rapid test will have a lower negative predictive value, producing a greater number of false negatives.

- *CDC - Influenza MMWR. http://www.cdc.gov/mmwr/preview/mmwrhtml/mm6332a3.htm*

#34

You are seeing a 25 year old male with HIV on HAART (atazanavir and indinavir) treatment. He had some routine labs drawn in follow-up and is found to have an elevated total bilirubin up to 5.0 mg/dL and the indirect portion being 4.5 mg/dL. The transaminases are normal, and the alkaline phosphatase is normal. What is the most likely etiology?

A. Hepatitis A, B, or C

B. Alcohol toxicity

C. Side effect of atazanavir that is likely benign

D. Cholangiopathy due to Cryptosporidium parvum

E. Direct toxic effect of HIV to the liver

#34

Answer: C

Atazanavir, along with indinavir, is associated with a benign, Gilbert's like-syndrome resulting in an increase in unconjugated bilirubin (indirect) which can cause an extensive hepatic evaluation in the ED if it is not recognized as a normal adverse effect. If the increase in bilirubin level is indirect and not direct bilirubin, generally no further evaluation is indicated for a patient receiving atazanavir.

- *Venkat A, et al. Care of the HIV-positive patient in the emergency department in the era of highly active antiretroviral therapy. Ann Emerg Med. 2008 Sep; 52(3): 274-85. full text*

#35

Rodent bites and scratches can transmit many diseases and bacteria, including all of the following EXCEPT:

A. Rat-bite fever

B. Leptospirosis

C. Tularemia

D. Rabies

E. Murine typhus and plague

#35

Answer: D

Rat-bite fever, leptospirosis, tularemia, sporotrichosis, murine typhus, and plague (Yersinia pestis) are just some of the many disease that are transmitted from rats to humans. Rabies, however, is not one of those diseases.

- *Rosen's Emergency Medicine - Concepts and Clinical Practice. 8th edition. 2013. Chapter 61: Mammalian Bites. 785-792.*
- *CDC - Plague. http://www.cdc.gov/plague/transmission/*

#36

The most common fungal pulmonary infection other than Pneumocystis jiroveci (PCP) in patients with AIDS is due to:

A. Cryptococcosis

B. Histoplasmosis

C. Coccidiomycosis

D. Aspergillosis

E. Nocardiosis

#36

Answer A

Cryptococcus neoformans is the most common fungal pathogen in patients with AIDS after pneumocystis jiroveci, typically causing infection in patients with CD4 counts < 100 cells/μliter. Radiographic findings are often nonspecific and may include consolidation, reticulonodular infiltrates and nodules. Diagnosis is with serum cryptococcal antigen assay.

- *Rosen's Emergency Medicine - Concepts and Clinical Practice. 8th edition. 2013. Chapter 132: HIV Infections and AIDS. 1758-1760.*

#37

True statements about Cryptococcus neoformans CNS infection include all of the following EXCEPT:

A. Most frequent initial symptoms include fever and headache.

B. Brainstem and basal ganglia are typical locations.

C. CT scan usually demonstrates significant changes consistent with Cryptococcus meningitis.

D. Cryptococcal CSF antigen is nearly 100% sensitive.

E. CSF india ink stain ranges from 60-80% sensitive.

#37

Answer C

C. neoformans is a fungal CNS infection that causes diffuse meningoencephalitis. It occurs in up to 10% of patients with HIV infection, but most commonly in those with CD4 counts < 100. The most frequent initial symptoms are fever and headache, often accompanied by nausea and vomiting. The brainstem and basal ganglia are typical locations. Lumbar puncture will almost always reveal elevated intracranial pressure. Definitive diagnosis relies on finding cryptococcal antigen in the CSF which is nearly 100% sensitive and specific; other diagnostic tests include India ink staining (60-80% sensitive), fungal culture (95% sensitive), and serum cryptococcal antigen (95% sensitive). All patients with a positive result on serum cryptococcal antigen assay should undergo lumbar puncture to rule out neurologic involvement. CT scan is not diagnostic.

- *Rosen's Emergency Medicine - Concepts and Clinical Practice. 8th edition. 2013. Chapter 132: HIV Infection and AIDS. 1761.*

#38

The most common cause of focal intracranial mass lesions in patients with HIV is:

A. Lymphoma

B. Cryptococcal infection

C. Cytomegalovirus

D. Toxoplasma gondii

E. Herpes Simplex Virus

#38

Answer D

T. gondii is the most common cause of focal intracranial mass lesions in patients with HIV, with an incidence of 3-4%. In most cases, symptomatic disease is a result of reactivation of latent infection. Common signs and symptoms include headache, fever, AMS, and seizures. Focal neurological deficits are found in up to 80% of cases, and serologic testing is NOT useful because up to 30% of the US population has antibodies to T. gondii.

Diagnosis is usually made by the presence of multiple subcortical lesions on CT scan. Note that T. gondii has a greater number of lesions with a predilection for the basal ganglia and corticomedullary area, whereas lymphoma tends to be singular lesions located in the periventricular matter or corpus callosum. Patients suspected of having Toxoplasmosis should be hospitalized and treated with pyrimethamine plus sulfadiazine, and folinic acid should be added to reduce the incidence of pancytopenia.

- *Rosen's Emergency Medicine - Concepts and Clinical Practice. 8th edition. 2013. Chapter 132: HIV Infection and AIDS. 1761.*

#39

You are seeing a patient in whom you are entertaining the diagnosis of tuberculous meningitis. True statements about this disease process include all of the following EXCEPT:

A. Treatment starts with a two-drug regimen for 6 months.

B. The classic triad of neuroradiologic findings in patients with TB meningitis consists of basal meningeal enhancement, hydrocephalus, and cerebral or brain stem infarction.

C. CSF protein is usually elevated.

D. The peak incidence of CNS TB is in newborn to 4 year old children.

E. TB cerebral involvement is most prominent at the base of the brain.

#39

Answer A

Treatment of tuberculosis meningitis consists of a four-drug regimen for 9 to 12 months, plus prednisone. TB meningitis commonly affects the brain stem and causes an associated vasculitis leading to aneurysm formation and hemorrhage. The CSF cell counts are elevated with a lymphocyte predominance. CSF cultures are only positive in 37% of cases.

- *Rosen's Emergency Medicine - Concepts and Clinical Practice. 8th edition. 2013. Chapter 135: Tuberculosis. 1820-1822.*

#40

You are seeing a 25 yo female with new-onset seizures. A head CT is obtained and demonstrates multiple calcifications, consistent with neurocysticercosis. TRUE statements about this include which of the following?

(Choose three answers.)

A. Cysticercosis is caused by the larval form of Taenia solium.

B. It is acquired by humans who eat pork containing the larval cysts.

C. The adult worm matures in the brain.

D. The diagnosis is made by brain biopsy.

E. Albendazole is the therapeutic agent of choice.

#40

Answer: A, B, and E

Neurocysticercosis is caused by T. solium, a worm that begins its life cycle in the small intestine but the larvae leave through the gut wall and can migrate to any organ. Most common sites are the CNS, muscle, and soft tissue. When the brain is involved, multiple larvae can form a cyst which induces fibrosis and results in calcifications, which will be visible on neuroimaging. Treatment for T. solium includes albendazole for active infections (based on stool analysis).

- *Rosen's Emergency Medicine - Concepts and Clinical Practice. 8th edition. 2013. Chapter 133: Parasitic Infections. 1777.*
- *CDC - Taeniasis. http://www.cdc.gov/parasites/taeniasis/biology.html*

#41

A 24 yo male presents to the ED saying that he had receptive anal intercourse without the use of a condom with a male partner who was known to have had sex with other men. He is also worried because many years ago she was not treated for a needlestick injury. TRUE statements about postexposure prophylaxis (PEP) for HIV include which of the following?

(Choose three answers.)

A. A case-control study in 1997 demonstrated that health care workers who received AZT after needlestick exposures were 81% less likely to undergo seroconversion to positivity for HIV.

B. The use of PEP does not assume that the person who was exposed to HIV is HIV negative.

C. The overall rate of HIV transmission through percutaneous inoculation through a needle is reported to be 0.3%.

D. The estimated risk of transmission from receptive anal intercourse is 50%.

E. The estimated transmission from receptive vaginal intercourse is 0.1-10%.

#41

Answer: A, C, and E

Providing PEP assumes that the patient with the exposure is HIV negative. A baseline negative HIV test should be documented along with PEP. Statement A, C and E are true. The estimated risk for receptive anal intercourse is 1 - 30%. The estimated risk of transmission associated with sharing needles for injection drug use is 0.67% per needle sharing contact. Overall risk after a needle stick is 0.3%. The generally recommended treatment is a four week dual nucleoside regimen such as zidovudine and lamivudine. However, adding a third agent such as ritonavir may improve efficacy.

- *Landovitz RJ, Currier JS. Postexposure prophylaxis for HIV infection. N Eng J Med. 2009 Oct 29; 361(18): 1768-75. full text*

#42

The overall rate of HIV transmission through percutaneous inoculation is widely reported to be 0.3%. Features of exposure that are associated with a higher rate of transmission include:

A. A needle that was used to cannulate a blood vessel in the source patient

B. Advanced HIV disease in the source patient

C. A deep needlestick

D. Visible blood on the surface of the instrument

E. All of the above

#42

Answer: E

All of the above exposure characteristics are associated with a higher rate of HIV transmission.

- *Landovitz RJ, Currier JS. Postexposure prophylaxis for HIV infection. N Engl J Med. 2009 Oct 29; 361(18): 1768-75. full text*

#43

A 28 yo male EM intern presents to the ED saying that he was stuck with a needle during an operative case on an HIV patient. TRUE statements about postexposure prophylaxis (PEP) for HIV include which of the following?

(Choose three answers.)

A. PEP should be initiated as rapidly as possible.

B. PEP should be continued for one week.

C. A three-drug PEP regimen based on nevirapine is thought to be ideal.

D. Reported rates of adherence to PEP is generally in the range of 70-80%.

E. PEP has become the standard of care for occupational exposures, but it remains controversial as a public health intervention for nonoccupational exposures.

#43

Answer: A, D, and E

PEP should be initiated as rapidly as possible and continued for 28 days, on the basis of Macaque primate studies. Two drug regimens of nucleosidases are commonly used with a protease inhibitor optionally added as a third drug to improve pharmacokinetics. Nevirapine is not recommended because its side effect profile includes hepatitis and serious cutaneous reactions when used in non-HIV infected patients. Statement D and E are true. Compliance can be increased with regular physician followup.

- *Landovitz RJ, Currier JS. Postexposure prophylaxis for HIV infection. N Engl J Med. 2009 Oct 29; 361(18): 1768-75. full text*

#44

You suspect that a 16 yo patient that you are currently evaluating with a several day history of fever, sore throat and malaise may have infectious mononucleosis (IM). TRUE statements about this disease process include which of the following?

(Choose three answers.)

A. IM is a clinical syndrome most commonly associated with reactivation or secondary Epstein Barr virus infection.

B. Over 95% of adults are infected with EBV.

C. Because economic and sanitary conditions have improved, pediatric EBV is less common, and incidence is greater in adolescents.

D. EBV transmission occurs primarily through the fecal-oral route.

E. Majority of patients with IM recover without significant complications.

#44

Answer: B, C and E

IM is a clinical syndrome that is caused by a primary EBV infection and more commonly during the first or second decade of life. Statements B, C, and E are true. EBV transmission occurs predominantly through exposure to infected saliva, often as a result of kissing, and less commonly by means of sexual transmission. The incubation period is estimated at 30-50 days.

. *Luzuriaga K, Sullivan JL. Infectious mononucleosis. N Eng J Med. 2010 May 27; 362(21): 1993-2000.*

#45

You suspect that a 16 yo patient that you are currently evaluating with a several day history of fever, sore throat and malaise may have infectious mononucleosis (IM). TRUE statements about the treatment of this disease process include which of the following?

A. Valacyclovir is recommended if the patient presents within the first 48 hours of symptom onset.

B. Corticosteroids should be used if the patient presents within the first 48 hours of symptom onset.

C. A return to contact sports may be permitted only after 6 months.

D. None of the above

E. All of the above

#45

Answer: D

The treatment of IM is largely supportive. Although there is great interest in developing antiviral regimens for treating IM, none have been definitively effective (valacyclovir and acyclovir have been tested). A Cochrane review that compared the effectiveness of corticosteroids with that of placebo concluded that there was insufficient evidence of a clinically relevant benefit to recommend steroids. Clinical experience suggests that steroids may be helpful in the management of more severe complications of IM, including pharyngitis and tonsillar swelling, hemolytic anemia, and thrombocytopenia. Given the rarity of splenic rupture after 3 weeks, a recent review concluded that patients can return to contact sports after 3 weeks if they are afebrile with symptom resolution.

- *Luzuriaga K, Sullivan JL. Infectious mononucleosis. N Engl J Med. 2010 May 27; 362(21): 1993-2000.*

#46

You suspect that a 16 yo patient that you are currently evaluating with a several day history of fever, sore throat and malaise may have infectious mononucleosis (IM). Which of the following statements about the diagnosis of this disease process is FALSE?

A. Infection with group A strep is the most common bacterial cause of pharyngitis, and distinguishing infection with group A strep from IM is important, since antibiotics may be warranted for group A strep.

B. Morbilliform rashes are common in patients with IM treated with amoxicillin or ampicillin (up to 95%).

C. Common laboratory findings include neutropenia.

D. The detection of at least 10% atypical lymphocytes has a sensitivity of 75% and specificity of 92% for the diagnosis of IM.

E. In the presence of IM symptoms, a positive heterophile (rapid monospot test) has a sensitivity of approximately 85% and a specificity of 94%.

#46

Answer: C

All of the statements are true except C. Patients with IM commonly have lymphocytosis (>50% leukocytes) with atypical lymphocytes. Note that while the heterophile antibodies can be helpful in young adults and adolescents, the monospot is positive in only 25-50% of children under 12 years of age. Also, heterophile antibody tests are usually negative in patients who have mononucleosis associated with CMV, human herpes virus, or toxoplasma.

- *Luzuriaga K, Sullivan JL. Infectious mononucleosis. N Engl J Med. 2010 May 27; 362(21): 1993-2000.*

#47

You are seeing a 52 yo diabetic female and she has recently noted erythema, swelling, and pain over the left foot. You are trying to determine whether this patient has osteomyelitis. Which of the following features are helpful in diagnosing the presence of lower extremity osteomyelitis in this patient?

(Choose two answers.)

A. The history and absence of a pulse

B. Ulcer area > 0.5 cm

C. Positive "probe to bone" test

D. ESR > 25 mm/h

E. Abnormal plain radiograph

#47

Answer: C and E

Osteomyelitis of the lower extremity is a common problem in patients with diabetes. The following are tests and their diagnostic values for identifying osteomyelitis.

An ulcer area larger than 2 cm

- Positive LR, 7.2; (95% CI, 1.1-49)
- Negative LR, 0.48; (95% CI, 0.31-0.76)

Positive "probe-to-bone" test result

- Positive LR, 6.4; (95% CI, 3.6-11)
- Negative LR, 0.39; (95% CI, 0.20-0.76)

Erythrocyte sedimentation rate > 70 mm/h

- Summary LR, 11; (95% CI, 1.6-79)

Abnormal plain radiograph

- Summary LR, 2.3; (95% CI, 1.6-3.3)

A positive MRI result

- Summary LR 3.8; (95% CI, 2.5-5.8).

A normal MRI result

- Summary LR, 0.14; (95% CI, 0.08-0.26).

The overall accuracy (ie, the weighted average of the sensitivity and specificity) of the MRI is 89% (95% CI, 83.0%-94.5%). In summary, large ulcers and the ability to probe to bone are the most useful physical exam findings. ESR is the most useful lab test. Temperature and white blood cell count are not helpful in the diagnosis of osteomyelitis in a diabetic. No single historical feature or physical examination reliably excludes osteomyelitis.

- *Butalia S, et al. Does this patient with diabetes have osteomyelitis of the lower extremity? JAMA. 2008 Feb 20; 299(7): 806-13. full text*

#48

You are evaluating a 70 year old male with a 3 week history of a cough. Which of the following features increases the likelihood of pertussis?

(Choose two answers.)

A. Presence of paroxysmal cough

B. Presence of posttussive emesis

C. Presence of inspiratory whoop

D. Fever

E. Nasal congestion and rhinorrhea

#48

Answer: B and C

According to a meta-analysis, by Cornia et al. the presence of posttussive emesis (LR, 1.8; 95% CI, 1.4-2.2) or inspiratory whoop (LR, 1.9; 95% CI, 1.4-2.6) increases the likelihood of pertussis.

Absence of paroxysmal cough (LR, 0.52; 95% CI, 0.27-1.0) or posttussive emesis (LR, 0.58; 95% CI, 0.44-0.77) reduced the likelihood. No studies evaluated combinations of findings. The authors conclude that the presence or absence of posttussive emesis or inspiratory whoop modestly change the likelihood of pertussis. Empiric antibiotics for pertussis should be based on clinical evaluation and time course of illness.

- *Cornia PB, et al. Does this coughing adolescent or adult patient have Pertussis? JAMA. 2010 Aug 25; 304(8): 890-6. full text*

#49

Regarding pertussis infection, which of the following statements is TRUE?

(Choose two answers.)

A. Infection with B pertussis is characterized by 3 phases: catarrhal, paroxysmal, and convalescent.

B. Incubation period for B pertussis is 1-2 days.

C. Symptoms of pertussis infection in previously immunized or infected adolescents and adults are variable and often atypical.

D. More than 90% of current cases of pertussis occur in children younger than 8 years of age.

E. When culturing for a nasopharyngeal specimen, one should swab the anterior nares and throat.

#49

Answer: A and C

The incubation period for pertussis is 7-10 days. Prior to the pertussis vaccine, 90% of reported pertussis cases were in children < 10 years of age. Currently, about half of reported cases occur in adolescents and adults. Posterior nasopharyngeal culture or antibody testing is used for diagnostic confirmation.

The CDC clinical definition of pertussis is a cough illness lasting 4 weeks or longer without other apparent cause with 1 or more of the following: paroxysms of coughing, inspiratory whoop or posttussive emesis.

Antibiotic treatment during the catarrhal phase may decrease the duration and severity of cough, but the diagnosis is rarely considered during this early phase in adolescents and adults. Although administering antibiotics later in the course of disease probably does not affect the course of symptoms, it is recommended to help reduce spread of infection. Persons may remain contagious for a month or longer. Azithromycin and clarithromycin have comparable efficacy and are better tolerated than erythromycin.

- *Cornia PB, et al. Does this coughing adolescent or adult patient have Pertussis? JAMA. 2010 Aug 25; 304(8): 890-6. full text*

- *CDC Pertussis http://www.cdc.gov/pertussis/clinical/*

#50

Which of the following patients with Lyme disease should get parenteral therapy?

(Choose two answers.)

A. A patient with Lyme disease and a cardiac conduction defect – first degree AV block with PR interval < 0.3 seconds

B. A patient who acquired the disease during pregnancy

C. A patient who has meningitis or encephalitis or a peripheral neuropathy

D. A patient with a high degree AV block with global ventricular impairment

E. All of the above

#50

Answer: C and D

Patients with late neurologic disease affecting the central or peripheral nervous system should be treated with ceftriaxone for 2-4 weeks. Patients with high degree block and ventricular dysfunction should be hospitalized for cardiac monitoring and treatment with parenteral antibiotics. Treatment for pregnant patients is identical to that for non-pregnant patients with the same disease manifestations except that doxycycline should be avoided. Pregnant patients usually receive amoxicillin. Most women give birth to normal infants despite documented Lyme borreliosis during their pregnancy.

- *Rosen's Emergency Medicine - Concepts and Clinical Practice. 8th edition. 2013. Chapter 134: Tick Borne Illness. 1786-1795.*

#51

You are seeing a patient who presents with hand pain and an open wound over the dorsal MCP joints after he punched someone in the mouth 5 days ago. It involves his dominant hand. TRUE statements about fight bites or clenched fist injury include which of the following?

(Choose two answers.)

A. Penetration of the joint occurs in up to 62% of wounds and up to 58% involve bone.

B. Presence of an extensor tendon laceration is highly predictive ofjoint penetration.

C. 100% of these injuries have cultures positive for Eikenella corrodens .

D. All ofthe above

#51

Answer: A and B

Eikenella corrodens, a facultatively anaerobic gram negative rod harbored in human dental plaque is found in 25-29% of clenched fist infections. The other two statements are correct.

- *Rosen's Emergency Medicine - Concepts and Clinical Practice. 8th edition. 2013. Chapter 59: Wound Management Principles. 764.*

#52

You are seeing a patient who had a generalized tonic-clonic seizure and bit the underside of his lower lip, resulting in a through-and-through laceration. TRUE statements about this injury include which of the following?

A. Wounds from the victim's own teeth may be considered bites.

B. Antibiotics are indicated.

C. Both of the above

D. None of the above

#52

Answer: C

Wounds from the victim's own teeth, usually a result from a fall or a seizure, may be considered bites. Wounds that involve only the mucosa or tongue have a low infection rate (0-12%), but through and through lacerations have an infection rate of up to 30% in the absence of prophylactic antibiotics. Organisms cultured from these infected wounds include Strep, Staph Aureus, Staph Epidermidis, Bacteroides, Corynebacterium, Neisseria, and Haemophilus.

- *Rosen's Emergency Medicine - Concepts and Clinical Practice. 8th edition. 2013. Chapter 59: Wound Management Principles. 764.*

#53

Lyme disease is due to transmission of B. burgdorferi through a tick bite; the initial site of infection is the skin at the site of the bite. After an incubation period of 1 week (range from 1 to 36 days), the spirochetes cause a gradually expanding infection in skin, called erythema migrans, which is the most characteristic clinical manifestation of Lyme disease. Shortly after disease onset, hematogenous spread can cause a variety of systemic signs and symptoms. Which of the following are the organ systems most commonly involved in secondary sites of infection?

(Choose three answers.)

A. Spleen

B. Subcutaneous tissue

C. Central nervous system

D. Heart

E. Joints

#53

Answer: C, D, and E

Organ systems commonly affected are the nervous system, heart, and joints. Less commonly, the eyes, liver, skeletal muscle, subcutaneous tissue, and spleen are infected. The most common neurologic manifestation of Lyme disease is a meningoencephalitis with superimposed symptoms of cranial neuropathy (bilateral Bell's Palsy), peripheral neuropathy, or radiculopathy.

Cardiac involvement may manifest as a conduction defect, myopericarditis, tachydysrhythmias, or ventricular impairment. Monoarticular or oligoarticular arthritis, primarily affecting large joints, especially the knee, may develop weeks to months after the onset of initial illness.

- *Rosen's Emergency Medicine - Concepts and Clinical Practice. 8th edition. 2013. Chapter 134: Tick Borne Illness. 1786-1795.*

#54

After a sexual assault, who should be offered prophylaxis in the ED for sexually transmitted infections?

A. Only in those who have a positive test after screening.

B. Only if the assailant is known to be positive for these illnesses.

C. All patients

#54

Answer: C

The CDC has published recommendations for treatment to prevent STI including Gonorrhea, Chlamydia, Trichomoniasis, Hepatitis B. If the assailant is known to be positive for HIV, the CDC recommends HIV postexposure prophylaxis.

- *CDC - Sexual Assault http://www.cdc.gov/std/treatment/2010/qanda/assault.htm*
- *CDC - Sexual Assault and STDs http://www.cdc.gov/std/treatment/2010/sexual-assault.htm*

#55

You are seeing a patient with HIV with a CD4 count of 50. He has not been compliant with his HAART therapy. TRUE statements about AIDS cholangiopathy include which of the following:

A. These disorders include bile duct stricture, papillary stenosis, and sclerosing cholangitis.

B. The pathophysiology is due to direct infection of the HIV virus in the biliary ducts.

C. Bilirubin is usually higher than in other disorders causing cholangitis.

D. Management includes removal of the bile duct, gallbladder and part of the liver.

#55

Answer: A

Biliary manifestations of advanced HIV disease, generally associated with CD4 counts < 200 may include any one of a group of disorders collectively referred to as AIDS cholangiopathy. These disorders include bile duct stricture, papillary stenosis, and sclerosing cholangitis. The diseases are related to infection with CMV, Cryptosporidium, Microsporidia, or Mycobacterium avium complex. Clinical presentations may be similar to that in other causes of cholangitis with fever and right upper quadrant pain.

Ultrasonography can identify bile duct strictures, thickening, or dilation. with treatment involving GI consult and surgical coordination for possible sphincterotomy, cholecystectomy and treatment of underlying infection.

- *Rosen's Emergency Medicine - Concepts and Clinical Practice. 8th edition. 2013. Chapter 90: Disorders of the Liver and Biliary Tract. 1204.*

#56

You are seeing a patient in whom you suspect spinal tuberculosis (Pott's disease). Which of the following statements is TRUE regarding this entity?

(Choose three answers.)

A. Fever and weight loss are present in the majority of patients.

B. Local pain is the most common symptom.

C. Diagnosis is often delayed.

D. There are no skeletal radiographic characteristics pathognomonic of TB.

E. Chest X-ray is a sensitive test for diagnosing skeletal TB.

#56

Answer: B, C, and D

In spinal TB, the most common symptom is local pain, which becomes more severe over several weeks to months, sometimes associated with muscle spasm and rigidity. Constitutional symptoms, fever, and weight loss may be present. Especially in countries where the incidence of tuberculosis is low, spinal tuberculosis is often delayed. Due to poor healthcare access in endemic areas, the diagnosis may be delayed and patients may present with cord compression at the time of diagnosis. There are no skeletal radiographic characteristics pathognomonic of TB. Chest radiography is not a sensitive test for the diagnosis of skeletal TB since more than 50% of such patients do not have evidence of active pulmonary disease.

. *Rosen's Emergency Medicine - Concepts and Clinical Practice. 8th edition. 2013. Chapter 136: Bone and Joint Infections. 1834-1836.*

#57

A 50 year old male who was recently released from prison reports that 2 weeks ago he had flu-like symptoms but now has 4 days of fevers as high as 104°F, chills, night sweats and cough productive of brown sputum. His exam is notable for absent breath sounds in the right lower lobe, and the chest X-ray demonstrates a large right-sided pleural effusion. Thoracentesis reveals pleural fluid with a pH of 7.1, glucose of 36, and LDH of 800. Gram stain of the pleural fluid demonstrates PMNs with intracellular gram-positive cocci in clusters. What is the next best step in management?

A. Chest tube and IV Unasyn

B. Chest tube and IV Vancomycin

C. Decortication by CT surgery

D. Decortication by CT surgery and IV Vancomycin

E. IV Vancomycin

#57

Answer: B

The patient has an empyema most likely secondary to MRSA, especially since he was incarcerated in the recent past (though MRSA is also rampant in the community) and had a preceding influenza like illness. In this case, chest tube placement and drainage is indicated along with initiation of antibiotics. Indications for drainage of an empyema include: pleural fluid pH < 7.2, glucose < 60, LDH> 600, and bacteria on gram stain. Empiric treatment with an antibiotic, such as IV vancomycin with a spectrum that covers MRSA would be appropriate. Final therapy decisions should be based on results of cultures and antimicrobial susceptibility testing. Unasyn does not have good activity against MRSA. Surgical decortication would be indicated for effusions with multiple loculations or those that have not responded to the tube drainage and for empyema at the organizing stage.

- *Rosen's Emergency Medicine - Concepts and Clinical Practice. 8th edition. 2013. Chapter 77: Pleural Disease. 994 - 996.*

MISCELLANEOUS

#1

Which of the following is NOT a legal standard or criteria for decision-making capacity?

A. Ability to communicate a choice

B. Understand the relevant information

C. Appreciate the situation and its consequences

D. Reason through treatment options

E. Score greater than 24 on the mini-mental status exam (MMSE)

#1

Answer: E

Legal standards for decision-making capacity for consenting to treatment vary across jurisdictions. At the core of the standards are a patient's ability to communicate a choice, understand the relevant information about the treatment or procedure, appreciate the medical consequences of the situation, and to reason through treatment choices. ANY physician who is aware of the relevant criteria should be able to assess a patient's competence. Psychiatric consultation may be helpful in particularly complex cases or when mental illness is present but are not required for assessing decisional capacity.

The Mini–Mental State Examination (MMSE) has been found to correlate with clinical judgments of incapacity, and it may have some use in identifying patients at the high and low ends of the range of capacity, especially among elderly persons with some degree of cognitive impairment. MMSE scores range from 0 to 30, with lower scores indicating decreasing cognitive function. No single cutoff score yields both high sensitivity and high specificity. MMSE scores of less than 19 are highly likely to be associated with incompetence. Studies vary in suggesting that scores of 23 to 26 or higher are strongly indicative of competence. However, incompetence is a legal designation, while capacity refers to a patient's mental soundness to make a decision regarding care.

- *Appelbaum PS. Assessment of Patients' Competence to Consent to Treatment. N Engl J Med. 2007 Nov 1; 357(18): 1834-40.*

#2

Regarding computed tomography, which of the following statements is FALSE?

A. It is estimated that more than 62 million CT scans per year are currently obtained in the United States, including at least 4 million for children.

B. The radiation doses to particular organs from any given CT study depend on many factors, which include, the tube current and scanning time, the size of the patient, the axial scan range, the scan pitch (the degree of overlap between adjacent CT slices), and the specific design of the scanner being used.

C. Cancer risks from radiation increase with increasing age.

D. There is direct evidence from epidemiologic studies that the greater the number of CT scans the greater the risk of cancer.

#2

Answer: C

Cancer risks from radiation exposure decrease with increasing age both because children have more years of life during which a potential cancer can develop (latency periods for solid tumors are typically decades) and because growing children are inherently more radiosensitive; they have a larger proportion of dividing cells.

- *Brenner DJ, et al. Computed Tomography – an increasing source of radiation exposure. N Engl J Med. 2007 Nov 29; 357(22): 2277-84. full text*

#3

Diagnostic errors are an important safety concern in the emergency department. Which of the following is NOT one of the leading causes of breakdowns in the diagnostic process?

A. Failure to order an appropriate test

B. Data entry problem

C. Failure to perform an adequate history or physical exam

D. Incorrect interpretation of a diagnostic test

E. Failure to order an appropriate consultation

#3

Answer: B

The leading breakdowns in the diagnostic process are failure to order an appropriate diagnostic test (58% of errors), failure to perform an adequate medical history or physical examination (42%), incorrect interpretation of a diagnostic test (37%), and failure to order an appropriate consultation (33%). The leading contributing factors to missed diagnoses are cognitive factors (96%), patient-related factors (34%), lack of appropriate supervision (30%), inadequate handoffs (24%), and excessive workload (23%). There is a median of two process breakdowns per missed diagnosis.

- *Kachalia A, et al. Missed and delayed diagnosis in the emergency department: a study of closed malpractice claims from 4 liability insurers. Ann Emerg Med. 2007 Feb; 49(2): 196-205.*

#4

Emergency physicians are best able to recognize adverse drug related events (ADRE) in the elderly population if the ADRE:

A. Was not serious

B. Was not related to the chief complaint

C. Was related to the chief complaint

D. Occurred in the last several weeks

E. None of the above

#4

Answer: C

Hohl, et al. examined the ability of emergency physicians (EPs) to recognize adverse drug-related events (ADREs) in elder patients presenting to the emergency department (ED). ADREs related to the patient's chief complaint were better recognized (91%; 95% CI = 74.1% to 100%) as compared with recognition of ADREs that were not associated with the chief complaint (32.1%; 95% CI = 14.8% to 49%).

The authors concluded that physician performance was good at identifying severe ADREs relating to patients' chief complaints but poor for identifying ADREs of lower severity as well as those unrelated to chief complaints.

- *LLSA 2007: Hohl CM, et al. Emergency physician recognition of adverse drug-related events in elder patients presenting to an emergency department. Acad Emerg Med. 2005 Mar; 12(3): 197-205.*

#5

Closed-claim reviews typically find fault with the thinking or behavior of individual physicians while ignoring equipment or process breakdowns that led to the actual error. Regarding diagnostic failures, which of the following statements is TRUE?

A. Both hindsight and outcome bias are present in quality assurance reviews.

B. In hindsight bias, those who know what happened after the fact overestimate what others who lacked that knowledge could have known.

C. Those who know the quality or desirability of the outcome, are biased towards judging the quality of the people involved in the error.

D. To decrease diagnostic failures, models of error correction should focus on actual daily care rather than ideal care.

E. All of the above

#5

Answer: E

Both hindsight and outcome bias are prominent in medical quality assurance and root cause analysis reviews. These biases make it hard for historical analyses to yield useful understanding of the adverse event or near miss. With hindsight bias, those who know what happened consistently overestimate what others who lacked that knowledge could have known. To the individuals performing the review, the adverse event appears as obviously avoidable. Reviewers who know the outcome of a case view the cues for a correct diagnosis as being much more evident, and events which were confusing during the treatment process become easily explainable.

Outcome bias is similar, where those who know the quality or desirability of the outcome use it to judge the quality of the process and people involved. For example, knowledge that a patient sustained an injury influences judgment about the quality of care.

Most patient safety reviews rely on a retrospective "error elimination" strategy that uses hindsight to identify and eliminate "causes" of "errors." Wears et al. suggest that a better approach would be to use experience to better understand current (and future) work and its inherent risks. If the circumstances leading to the adverse events can be understood, then there can be lasting improvements to clinical practice which prevents further errors.

- *LLSA 2009: Wears RL, et al. Replacing hindsight with insight: toward better understanding of diagnostic failures. Ann Emerg Med. 2007; 49(2): 206-209. full text*

#6

Certain classes of minors are legally competent to provide consent for treatment. Which of the following fall into this category?

A. Minors who live on their own

B. Minors who are in the US military

C. Minors who are pregnant

D. Minors who are already parents

E. All of the above

#6

Answer: E

All of the above are considered emancipated minors. In addition, minors who present for treatment for drug rehabilitation, sexually transmitted diseases, or pregnancy may also legally consent to treatment.

- *Harwood-Nuss' Clinical Practice of Emergency Medicine. 5th edition. 2010. Chapter 366: Ethical Issues. 1677.*

#7

Regarding refusal of care, which of the following statements is FALSE?

A. Competency is a legal concept, and under the law, all adult persons are presumed to be legally competent.

B. A person may be declared legally incompetent only in the setting of a formal judicial proceeding in which a judge hears testimony from expert witnesses, usually psychiatrists or neurologists.

C. Capacity is a legal concept, and under the law, all adult persons are presumed to have decision making capacity.

D. To provide a valid refusal, the patient must be competent to do so and possess adequate decision making capacity.

E. Minors, with some exceptions, are legally incompetent and may neither refuse or consent to treatment.

#7

Answer: C

Capacity is a medical concept and is the basis by which physicians determine whether patients are capable of understanding the nature of their disease and the ramifications of accepting or refusing treatment. The physician should ascertain the decision making capacity of every patient who refuses treatment by performing a mental status examination and by inquiring regarding whether the patient has a full understanding of the nature of the illness and the risks associated with forgoing treatment. Patients who have adequate decision making capacity and who understand the treatment recommendations of their physicians may refuse treatment, even if their refusal may result in death

- *Harwood-Nuss' Clinical Practice of Emergency Medicine. 5th edition. 2010. Chapter 366: Ethical Issues. 1674-1677.*

#8

Which of the following is NOT one of the elements of a professional liability action (medical malpractice claim) against an emergency physician?

A. The emergency physician owed a patient a duty of reasonable care.

B. The physician breached that duty of reasonable care.

C. The emergency physician is board certified.

D. There is a causal connection between the physician's conduct and the resulting injury to the plaintiff.

E. There is an actual injury to the patient.

#8

Answer: C

The four elements of a professional liability action against an emergency physician are duty, breach, causation, and damages. Generic allegations against emergency physicians in professional liability actions (medical malpractice claims) are:

1. Failure to order a diagnostic test
2. Failure to properly interpret the results of a test
3. Failure to obtain a consult
4. Failure to admit a patient

- *Harwood-Nuss' Clinical Practice of Emergency Medicine. 5th edition. 2010. Chapter 367: Legal Issues. 1679.*

#9

Which of the following is NOT covered under GENERAL CONSENT – a type of consent emergency department clerical personnel obtain when a patient signs in?

A. Triage

B. Taking vital signs

C. Connecting patient to a monitor

D. Obtaining a history and physical

E. All of the above are covered under general consent

#9

Answer: E

In addition, performing basic diagnostic tests (lab tests, electrocardiograms, and X-rays), and initiating non-invasive or minimally invasive treatment are all activities covered under a general consent. A general consent is NOT informed, and very little if any discussion about the nature of the patient's illness or diagnostic and treatment plan occurs with this type of consent.

- *Harwood-Nuss' Clinical Practice of Emergency Medicine 5th edition. 2010. Chapter 367: Legal Issues. 1680.*

#10

Regarding informed consent, which of the following is TRUE?

A. Informed consent is a process, not just a piece of signed paper.

B. Physician should disclose the indications for the treatment.

C. Physician should disclose the risks associated with the treatment.

D. Physician should disclose any alternative treatments.

E. All of the above

#10

Answer: E

In addition to the above, the physician should describe the risks associated with the alternative treatments. During the process of obtaining informed consent, the patient should be given an opportunity to ask questions. The act of merely asking a patient to sign a standardized form without the above discussion is not consistent with a properly executed informed consent.

- *Harwood-Nuss' Clinical Practice of Emergency Medicine 5th edition. 2010. Chapter: 367: Legal Issues. 1680.*

#11

The "emergency exception to the general consent rule" allows emergency medical personnel, including prehospital providers to provide necessary stabilizing treatment to patients who are unable to provide consent as a result of their conditions. The requirements that must be met for the "emergency privilege" to apply include which of the following?

A. Patient must be unconscious or without capacity to make a decision.

B. No one legally authorized to act as an agent for the patient is available.

C. Time must be of the essence, such that any delay would subject the person to a risk of bodily injury or death.

D. Under the circumstances, a reasonable person would consent.

E. All of the above

#11

Answer: E

All of these requirements must be met. If there is any doubt regarding the emergency consent doctrine, it is best to err on the side of treatment and obtain the patient's or surrogate consent later.

- *Harwood-Nuss' Clinical Practice of Emergency Medicine 5th edition. 2010. Chapter 367: Legal Issues. 1680.*

#12

Regarding the Emergency Medical Treatment and Active Labor Act (EMTALA), which of the following is FALSE?

A. EMTALA's first mandate is that all individuals who present to the ED requesting emergency care must receive a Medical Screening Exam (MSE) to determine whether an emergency medical condition exists.

B. EMTALA defines a medical screening exam as triage.

C. A MSE must be performed to the same extent for the same complaint for individuals who have insurance and those who do not.

D. If the individual is admitted for treatment, the MSE requirement ends.

E. MSE may not be delayed to determine whether the individual has insurance coverage.

#12

Answer: B

An MSE is not triage, because it must include ancillary services. EMTALA does not define an MSE but does state that the MSE is based on the ED's capability, including ancillary services, such as diagnostic tests and specialty consultations typically available in the ED. In cases in which an individual is not seeking emergency care, a brief questioning by qualified personnel regarding the reason the individual presented to the ED will fulfill the MSE requirement.

. *Harwood-Nuss' Clinical Practice of Emergency Medicine 5th edition. 2010. Chapter 368: Regulatory Issues. 1684-1685.*

#13

A researcher/investigator decides to examine cigarette smoking exposure in a group of ED patients with pneumonia and those without pneumonia. Which of the following types of study designs best describes this?

A. Cohort study

B. Cross-sectional study

C. Case-control study

D. Randomized controlled trial

E. None of the above

#13

Answer: C

In a case-control design, the investigator compares a group of subjects who have a disease or condition with another group of subjects who do not. In a cohort study, a group of subjects is followed over time. In cross-sectional studies, observations are made on a single occasion.

- *Hulley SB, et al. Designing Clinical Research. 2nd edition. Philadelphia, PA: Lippincott Williams & Wilkins; 2001.*

#14

Suppose an investigator finds an association between coffee drinking and myocardial infarction (MI). Before concluding that coffee drinking is a cause of MI, which of the following rival explanations must be considered?

A. Random error

B. Bias

C. Effect-cause (having an MI causes people to drink coffee)

D. Confounding

E. All of the above

#14

Answer: E

Random error (chance) and systematic error (bias) can contribute to spurious associations between coffee drinking and MI (ie. associations are found only in the study, and not in the general population). Two other possibilities include effect-cause relationship (ex.having an MI makes people drink more coffee) and confounding factor (ex. some third factor such as cigarette smoking is a cause of MI and is associated with coffee drinking).

- *Hulley SB, et al. Designing Clinical Research. 2nd edition. Philadelphia, PA: Lippincott Williams & Wilkins; 2001.*

#15

Select the INCORRECT statement below regarding relative and absolute risk:

A. Relative risk reduction is the percentage reduction in events in the treated event rate compared to the control group event rate.

B. The number needed to treat is the inverse of the relative risk reduction.

C. The number needed to treat is a useful measure of benefit, as it tells you the absolute number of patients who need to be treated to prevent one bad outcome.

D. Relative risk is a ratio of the risk in the experimental group to the risk in the control group.

#15

Answer: B

The number needed to treat is the inverse of the absolute risk reduction, which is the absolute difference between the control and experimental group. The absolute risk reduction is a more clinically relevant measure to use than the relative risk reduction. Relative risk reduction "factors out" the baseline risk, so that small differences in risk can seem significant when compared to a small baseline risk.

- *Spitalnic S. Risk Assessment I: Relative Risk and Absolute Risk Reduction. Hospital Physicians. 2005; 43-46.*

#16

Which of the following is FALSE?

A. Positive predictive value is the proportion of people with a positive test who have disease.

B. Post-test probability is the proportion of people with disease who have a positive test.

C. Prevalence is the baseline risk of a disorder in the population of interest.

D. Specificity is the proportion of people free of a disease who have a negative test.

E. Spectrum bias is the bias caused by a study population whose disease profile does not reflect that of the intended population (for example, they have more severe forms of the disorder).

#16

Answer: B

Post-test probability is the probability that a patient has the disorder of interest after the test result is known. Sensitivity is the proportion of people with disease who have a positive test.

- *Spitalnic S. Test Properties I: Sensitivity, Specificity, and Predictive Values. Hospital Physicians. 2004; 27-31.*

#17

Which of the following is FALSE?

A. Publication bias is a bias in a systematic review caused by incompleteness of the search, such as omitting non-English language sources, or unpublished trials (inconclusive trials are less likely to be published than conclusive ones, but are not necessarily less valid).

B. Selection bias is a bias in assignment or selection of patients for a study that arises from study design rather than by chance.

C. A sensitivity analysis is the process of testing how sensitive a result would be to changes in factors such as baseline risk, susceptibility, the patients' best and worst outcomes, etc.

D. Recall bias is bias due to cases being missed because they have not had time to develop or are too mild to be detected at the time of the study.

E. A reference standard is a diagnostic test used in trials to confirm presence or absence of the target disorder.

#17

Answer: D

Recall bias is a systematic error due to the differences in accuracy or completeness of recall to memory of past events or experiences. Neyman bias is bias due to cases being missed because they have not had time to develop or are too mild to be detected at the time of the study. All of the other statements are true.

- *Raphael K. Recall bias: a proposal for assessment and control. Int J Epidemiol. 1987; 16(2): 167-170.*

#18

Diagnosis-related errors are often difficult to understand; however, progress towards better understanding will take into account hindsight and outcome bias. TRUE statements include:

A. Hindsight bias occurs when a reviewer overestimates what others should have known.

B. Outcome bias changes perception ofhe quality of the case based on prior knowledge ofthe bad outcome.

C. Both ofthe above are true.

D. Neither ofthe above are true

#18

Answer: C

Hindsight bias occurs when a reviewer overestimates what others should have known at the time of case presentation. Reviewers of a complex case see the earlier history as being much more obvious and conclude that the information should have led to the known diagnosis. However, a diagnosis judged in hindsight to be wrong might have been based on a sound medical decision-making at presentation. Outcome bias affects the judgment of the quality of the case based on the knowledge of the bad outcome in the absence of a causal relationship.

- *LLSA 2009: Wears RL, et al. Replacing hindsight with insight: toward better understanding of diagnostic failures. Ann Emerg Med. 2007; 49(2): 206-209. full text*

#19

According to an Institute of Medicine report, which was created to summarize the current state of emergency care, which of the following is FALSE?

A. Although the number of patient visits increased from 90 million to 114 million, 425 EDs closed nationally between 1993 to 2003.

B. There is a lack of EMS and disaster preparedness.

C. Although 27% of all ED visits are pediatric, the majority of EDs are ill equipped or staffed to handle pediatric emergencies.

D. There is an excess of on-call specialists.

E. 23-hour observation units should be created to decrease crowding and unnecessary admissions.

#19

Answer: D

Due to decreasing reimbursement for ED services, increased liability and malpractice premiums associated with caring for ED patients and the disruption to private practice and family life that on-call coverage requires, there is a shortage of on-call specialists in most EDs. According to EMTALA, a hospital that offers specialist service to inpatients must also offer these services to ED patients.

- *LLSA 2008: Institute Of Medicine. IOM report: The Future of Emergency Care in the United States Health System. Acad Emerg Med. 2006 Oct; 13(10): 1081-5.*

#20

Which of the following patients does not warrant monitoring with telemetry after admission to the hospital?

A. AICD firing

B. Type II and complete heart block

C. Decompensated heart failure

D. Acute cerebrovascular accident

E. Massive blood transfusion

F. All of the above warrant monitoring

#20

Answer: F

In addition to the above, those with a prolonged QT interval with ventricular arrhythmias and acute coronary syndrome patients warrant monitoring. Non-intensive telemetry units are utilized for monitoring patients at risk for life-threatening dysrhythmias and sudden death. Physicians often use monitored beds for patients who might only require frequent nursing care.

When 70% of the top 10 diseases admitted through the emergency department (ED) are clinically indicated for telemetry, hospitals with limited resources will be overwhelmed. This causes increased boarding in the ED. There is evidence for monitoring in patients admitted for implantable cardioverter-defibrillator firing, type II and complete atrioventricular block, prolonged QT interval with ventricular arrhythmia, decompensated heart failure, acute cerebrovascular event, acute coronary syndrome, and massive blood transfusion.

Monitoring is beneficial for selected patients with syncope, gastrointestinal hemorrhage, atrial tachyarrhythmias, and uncorrected electrolyte abnormalities. Telemetry is not indicated for patients requiring minor blood transfusions, low risk chest pain patients with normal electrocardiography, and stable patients receiving anticoagulation for pulmonary embolism.

- *LLSA 2009: Chen EH and Hollander JE. When do patients need admission to a telemetry bed? J Emerg Med. 2007; 33(1): 53-60. full text*

#21

In November 2006, the National Quality Forum endorsed new safe-practice guidelines on the disclosure of serious unanticipated outcomes to patients. The key elements of safe practice for disclosing unanticipated outcomes to patients includes all of the following EXCEPT:

A. Write a letter to hospital administration about the event.

B. Provide facts about the event to the patient.

C. Express regret for unanticipated outcome to the patient.

D. Give formal apology to the patient if unanticipated outcome was caused by an error or system failure.

E. Integrate disclosure, patient-safety and risk-management activities.

#21

Answer: A

The key elements of the safe practice for disclosing unanticipated outcomes to patients include

1. Providing facts about the event to the patient
2. Expressing regret for the unanticipated outcome
3. Giving a formal apology if there is a system failure or an error

At the institutional level, key elements include

1. Encouraging disclosure
2. Patient safety and risk management personnel
3. Establishing a disclosure support system
4. Using performance improvement tools to track and enhance disclosure

- *Gallagher TH, et al. Disclosing Harmful Medical Errors to patients. 2007 Jun 28; 356(26): 2713-9. full text*

#22

A 75-year-old woman with type 2 diabetes mellitus with osteomyelitis and a gangrenous midfoot is recommended to undergo an amputation. The patient states that she does not want to live without a foot and would rather die then undergo the procedure. She was rational yet difficult in the emergency department but while on the floor was noted to be intermittently confused with her surroundings. In regard to assessing her ability to refuse the procedure, there are four generally accepted legal standards for decision-making standards for consent and refusal for treatment. Which of the following is NOT one of these?

A. Patient must be hemodynamically stable.

B. Patient must be able to communicate his/her choice.

C. Patient must understand the relevant information.

D. Patient must understand the medical consequences ofthe situation.

E. Patient must be able to reason about the treatment choices.

#22

Answer: A

Decision-making capacity requires:

1. The ability to communicate a choice
2. To understand the relevant information
3. To appreciate the medical consequences of the situation
4. To reason about treatment choices.

Although the patient may be acting in a manner against recommendations of the treating physicians, if she can demonstrate the above four requirements for decisional capacity then she should be considered competent to make a treatment decision. If there is concern regarding her cognitive abilities, then one of the many screening tools or a psychiatric consultation can be helpful. However, any physician, not just psychiatrists can assess decisional capacity.

- *Appelbaum PS. Assessments of patients' competence to consent to treatment. N Engl J Med. 2007 Nov 1; 357(18): 1834-40.*

#23

You have committed a medication error while caring for a patient. In terms of what is now recommended by the National Quality Forum, the content to be disclosed to the patient includes which of the following elements?

A. Facts about the event

B. Presence of error or system failure, if known

C. Results of event analysis

D. Regret for unanticipated outcome

E. All of the above

#23

Answer: E

Disclosure of unanticipated outcomes to patients is now a core component of high-quality health care. Traditionally, communication with patients about unanticipated outcomes has been handled by risk managers who sought to minimize malpractice claims. Framing disclosure as a piece of improved patient safety allows for system improvements to take place while also encouraging the risk-management, patient-safety, and quality programs to work together.

- *Gallagher TH, et al. Disclosing harmful medical errors to patients. N Engl J Med. 2007 Jun 28; 356(26):2713-9. full text*

#24

In a randomized controlled trial comparing absorbable sutures for laceration closure vs. non-absorbable nylon sutures, which of the following differences were noted?

A. Infection rates

B. Dehiscence rates

C. Need for surgical revision

D. Comfort

E. None of the above

#24

Answer: E

Karounis H, et al. conducted a pediatric emergency department (1999-2001) based trial where patients 1-18 years of age with lacerations < 12 hours old were randomized into two groups:

1. Absorbable plain gut sutures (group A)
2. Non-absorbable nylon sutures (group NA)

Exclusion criteria were the following: wounds that could be approximated by tissue adhesives, animal/human bites, gross contamination, puncture/crush wounds, wounds crossing joints, lacerations of tendon/nerve/cartilage, collagen vascular disease, immunodeficiency, diabetes mellitus, bleeding disorder, and scalp lacerations.

A score of 6/6 was considered optimal. The study nurse also noted the presence of infection and dehiscence. The patients were then seen by a single blinded plastic surgeon at four or five months who evaluated the wound using a previously validated visual analog scale of cosmesis (VAS). In addition, the surgeon repeated the WES and assessed the need for surgical scar revision.

- *Karounis H, et al. A randomized controlled trial comparing long-term cosmetic outcomes of traumatic pediatric lacerations repaired with absorbable plain gut versus nonabsorbable nylon sutures. Acad Emerg Med. 2004; 11(7): 730-735.*

#25

Which of the following types of radiographic studies exposes the studied relevant organ to the most radiation?

A. PA chest radiograph - lung

B. Adult CT of the head - brain

C. Adult CT of the abdomen – stomach

D. Neonatal CT of the abdomen – stomach

E. Mammogram – breast

#25

Answer: D

Pediatric patients have thinner torsos and less abdominal fat, and therefore have less shielding from radiation exposure. Pediatric organs exposed to radiation during a CT receive higher doses than an adult receiving a CT. The mAs of the CT scan can be reduced in pediatric patients. As CT scanning technology advances, the scans will be able to perform with similar quality images while using less radiation.

- *Brenner DJ, et al. Computed tomography – an increasing source of radiation exposure. N Engl J Med. 2007 Nov 29; 357(22): 2277-84. http://bit.ly/kaji-increasing-rad*

#26

Regarding exposure to radioactive iodine and treatment with potassium iodide (KI), which of the following statements is TRUE?

A. Potassium iodide is the drug of choice to prevent thyroid uptake of radioiodine.

B. Potassium iodide provides no protection from external irradiation.

C. Potassium iodide must be administered within a few hours of exposure to confer its thyroid protective benefits.

D. Children are more vulnerable to the effects of radioiodine than adults.

E. Potassium iodide in the setting of acute radioiodine exposure is rarely indicated for adults older than 40 and only if there is a projected thyroid dose of 5 Gy or greater.

F. All of the above

#26

Answer: F

Potassium iodide is the drug of choice to prevent thyroid uptake of radio-iodines, but it provides no protection from external irradiation. It must be administered within a few hours of exposure to confer its thyroid-protective benefits and may be especially beneficial in children.

Potassium iodide therapy in the setting of acute radioiodine exposure is rarely indicated for adults older than 40 years and generally only if there is a projected thyroid dose of 5 Gy or greater. In pediatric populations, therapy should be initiated when exposure to as little as 10 mGy of radiation. The side effects of potassium iodide, however, include rashes, allergic reactions, and gastrointestinal symptoms. KI administered to people with underlying thyroid disease increases their risk of iodine-induced thyroid dysfunction.

- *Koenig KL, et al. Medical treatment of radiological casualties: current concepts. Ann Emerg Med. 2005 Jun; 45(6): 643-52. full text*

Term	Definition
A. Sensitivity	1. The number of true positives and true negatives divided by the total number of observations.
B. Specificity	2. A measure of the odds of having a disease relative to the prior probability of the disease. The estimate is independent of the disease prevalence.
C. Number needed to treat	3. The number of patients with a positive test who have a disease divided by all patients who have the

	disease.
D. Positive predictive value	4. The ability of a study to detect a true difference.
E. Negative predictive value	5. The reciprocal of the absolute risk reduction (the absolute adverse event rate for placebo minus the absolute adverse event rate for treated patients).
F. Likelihood ratio	6. The incidence in exposed individuals divided by the incidence in unexposed individuals.
G. Odds ratio	7. Equals the sum of observations divided by the number of observations.
H. Risk ratio	8. Equals the odds that an individual with a specific condition has been exposed to a risk factor divided by the odds that a control has been exposed.
I. Mode	9. The observation that occurs most frequently.
J. Mean	10. Refers to the extent to which repeated measurements of a relatively stable phenomenon fall closely to each other.
K. Median	11. The observation in the middle when all observations are ordered from smallest to largest.
L. Accuracy	12. The probability of incorrectly concluding that there was no statistically

	significant difference in a dataset. This error often reflects insufficient power of the study.
M. Power	13. Number of patients who have a negative test and do not have the disease divided by the number of patients who do not have the disease.
N. Type II error	14. Represents the likelihood that a patient with a positive test has the disease.
O. Reliability	15. Represents the likelihood that a patient who has a negative test does not have the disease.
P. Validity	16. The extent to which an observation reflects the "truth" of the phenomenon being measured.
Q. Standard deviation	17. The probability of incorrectly concluding that there is a statistically significant difference in a dataset.
R. Type I error	18. Measures the variability of data around the mean. It provides information on how much variability can be expected among individuals within a population.

#27 Match the epidemiological term with the correct definition.

#27

Answers:

A-3

B-13

C-5

D-14

E-15

F-2

G-8

H-6

I-9

J-7

K-11

L-1

M-4

N-12

O-10

P-16

Q-18

R-17

#28

You are seeing a patient who is 70 years old and has mild dementia. He is refusing to stay in the hospital for an evaluation of his chest pain. To determine whether he has capacity to make a decision, which of the following would be most helpful?

A. MMSE

B. Psychiatry consult

C. Ethics consult

D. Social work consult

E. None of the above

#28

Answer: A

MMSE scores range from 0 to 30, with lower scores indicating decreasing cognitive function. No single cutoff score yields both high sensitivity and high specificity. MMSE scores of less than 19 are highly likely to be associated with decreased decisional capacity.

Psychiatric consultation may be helpful in particularly complex cases or when mental illness is present. The Mini–Mental State Examination (MMSE) has been found to correlate with clinical judgments of incapacity, and it may have some use in identifying patients at the high and low ends of the range of capacity, especially among elderly persons with some degree of cognitive impairment.

- *Appelbaum PS. Assessment of Patients' Competence to Consent to Treatment. N Engl J Med. 2007 Nov 1; 357(18): 1834-40. full text*

#29

Regarding foreign bodies, which of the following statements is TRUE?

A. Esophageal foreign bodies are usually oriented in the sagittal plane.

B. Tracheal foreign bodies are usually oriented in the coronal plane.

C. Unresolving sinusitis despite appropriate antibiotic therapy should alert the emergency physician to the possibility of a nasal foreign body.

D. Esophageal foreign bodies are typically found at one of three constriction locations, one of which is in the oropharynx.

E. None of the above.

#29

Answer: C

Classically, esophageal foreign bodies usually are oriented in the coronal plane, whereas airway objects usually are oriented in the sagittal plane, parallel to the tracheal rings. Esophageal foreign bodies typically are found at one of 3 constriction locations:

1. Proximal esophagus at the level of the cricopharyngeal muscle and thoracic inlet
2. Midesophagus at the level of the aortic arch and carina
3. Distal esophagus just proximal to the esophagogastric junction.

The classic teaching of tracheal and esophageal foreign bodies is not absolute. Esophageal foreign bodies can certainly be oriented sagittally and tracheal foreign bodies coronally.

- Rosen's Emergency Medicine - Concepts and Clinical Practice. 8th edition. 2013. Chapter 60: Foreign Bodies. 776-778.

- *Schlesinger AE, Crowe JE. Sagittal orientation of ingested coins in the esophagus in children. AJR Am J Roentgenol. 2011 Mar; 196(3): 670-2. full text*

#30

You are now caring for a number of patients in the ED, all of whom are older than 65 years of age. TRUE statements about the older population include which of the following:

(Choose two answers.)

A. Compared to all other age groups, patients over the age of 65 years have a greater mortality risk during their hospitalization.

B. A higher ED lactate is associated with a greater mortality in patients over 65 yo with an infection, but not in those without an infection.

C. Lactate is linearly related to 30-day, 60-day, and 90-day mortality.

D. Lactate has a greater magnitude of association with mortality than creatinine, but not as great an association as leukocyte count has with mortality.

#30

Answer: A and C

In a retrospective cohort study performed at two urban teaching hospitals involving 1,655 older ED patients (age ≥ 65 years) over a 3-year period (2004-2006) who had serum lactate measured prior to admission higher ED lactate values were associated with greater mortality regardless of the presence or absence of infection. Infection status was determined by review of ICD-9 admission diagnosis codes. Mortality during hospitalization was determined by review of inpatient records. Mortality at 30 and at 60 days was determined using a state death registry.

In patients with infections, increasing serum lactate values of ≥ 2.0 mmol/L were linearly associated with relative risk (RR) of mortality during hospitalization (RR=1.9 to 3.6 with increasing lactate), at 30 days (RR=1.7 to 2.6), and at 60 days (RR=1.4 to 2.3) when compared to patients with serum lactate levels of <2.0 mmol/L. In patients without infections, a similar association was observed (RR=1.1 to 3.9 during hospitalization, RR=1.2 to 2.6 at 30 days, RR=1.1 to 2.4 at 60 days). In both groups of patients, serum lactate had a greater magnitude of association with mortality than either leukocyte count or serum creatinine.

- *Del Portal DA, et al. Emergency department lactate is associated with mortality in older adults admitted with and without infections. Acad Emerg Med. 2010 Mar; 17(3): 260-8.*

#31

Regarding ED crowding and boarding to inpatient hallways vs. boarding in the ED, which of the following is TRUE?

(Choose three answers.)

A. ED crowding negatively affects care, as it reduces access to EMS and is associated with delays in care for cardiac and stroke patients, as well as with pneumonia.

B. ED crowding is associated with an increase in patient mortality and prolonged patient transport time, inadequate pain management and decreased physician job satisfaction.

C. When comparing ED boarded patients that are transferred to inpatient hallways versus patients admitted to standard beds, in-hospital mortality was higher for those transferred to inpatient hallways.

D. ICU transfers were higher in the ED boarder patients admitted to the inpatient hallways than among patients admitted to standard beds.

E. There is widespread resistance to boarding of admitted patients to inpatient hallways, because of concern for greater risk of poor outcomes and harm.

#31

Answer: A, B, and E

According to a 4 year retrospective cohort study conducted at Stony Brook University of 55,062 admitted ED patients, there were 1,798 deaths. Of all admissions, 2,042 (4%) went to a hallway; 53,020 went to a standard bed. Patients admitted to standard and hallway beds were similar in age (median [interquartile range] 55 years [37 to 72 years] and 54 years [41 to 70 years], respectively) and sex (48.2% and 50% female patients, respectively). The median (interquartile range) times from ED triage to actual admission in patients admitted to standard and hallway beds were 426 minutes (306 to 600 minutes) and 624 (439 to 895 minutes) minutes, respectively (P<.001). Median ED census at triage was lower for standard bed admissions than for hallway patients (44 [33 to 53] versus 50 [38 to 61], respectively, P<.001).

In-hospital mortality rates were higher among patients admitted to standard beds (2.6%; 95% confidence interval [CI] 2.5% to 2.7%) than among patients admitted to hallway beds (1.1%; 95% CI 0.7% to 1.7%). ICU transfers were also higher in the standard bed admissions (6.7% [95% CI 6.5% to 6.9%] versus 2.5% [95% CI 1.9% to 3.3%]). Transfer of ED-boarded admitted patients to an inpatient hallway occurred during high ED census and waiting times for admission but did not appear to result in patient harm.

- *Viccellio A, et al. The association between transfer of emergency department boarders to inpatient hallways and mortality: a 4-year experience. Ann Emerg Med. 2009 Oct; 54(4): 487-91.*

#32

Regarding older patients in the emergency department, which of the following statements is TRUE?

A. Older patients are at increased risk of ED return visits, hospitalization, and death.

B. Older people (>65 years) account for 1-2% of all ED visits.

C. Delirium in the ED is recognized with high sensitivity and specificity.

D. Depression is rare in the older patient population.

E. Motor vehicle crashes are the main cause of ED admissions for elderly patients.

#32

Answer: A

Overall, older people (>65 years) account for 12-24% of all ED visits and have a greater frequency of return visits, hospitalization and death. Impaired mental status occurs in nearly 25% of older patients as a result of dementia or delirium. Unfortunately, delirium is recognized in the ED with a high specificity (98-100%) but a fairly low sensitivity (16-35%). Depression may be present in up to 1/3 of older ED patients and may interfere with the clinical presentation of acute medical disorders. Falls are the main cause of ED admissions for elderly patients (15-30%).

- *Samaras N, et al. Older patients in the emergency department: a review. Ann Emerg Med. 2010 Sep;56(3): 261-9. full text*

#33

Regarding older patients in the ED, which of the following statements is TRUE?

(Choose two answers.)

A. The majority of the elderly population who have acute myocardial infarction present with a chief complaint of TYPICAL chest pain.

B. Likelihood of treatment with aspirin and beta-blockers after MI decreases by 15 and 21% respectively for every 10 years of increasing age after 65 years.

C. There is a validated screening method for detecting polypharmacy and adverse drug effects in the elderly.

D. CAGE has been validated as a screening questionnaire among the elderly, and thus the majority of elderly current alcohol abusers are detected in the ED.

E. Compared with that of younger patients, older patients who have abdominal pain have mortality rates that are 6 to 8 times higher and surgery rates that are increased 2-fold.

#33

Answer: B and E

The presentation of acute myocardial infarction in older patients is frequently atypical, presenting as shortness of breath, syncope, nausea and vomiting, and falls. In 2005, older emergency department patients with acute myocardial infarction were shown to receive lower quality of care than younger patients. Adverse drug effects lead to 11% of ED visits in patients older than 65 years of age. Unfortunately, no validated screening method exists, and obtaining an accurate list of drugs is frequently difficult. Only 21% of elderly alcohol abusers are detected in the ED. No validated screening instrument for substance abuse in geriatric patients is available.

- *Samaras N, et al. Older patients in the emergency department: a review. Ann Emerg Med. 2010 Sep;56(3): 261-9. full text*

- *Magid DJ, et al. Older emergency department patients with acute myocardial infarction receive lower quality of care than younger patients. Ann Emerg Med. 2005 Jul; 46(1): 14-21.*

#34

Regarding the Identification of Seniors at Risk tool (ISAR) for screening high-risk older patients in the ED, which of the following are factors that increase risk of an adverse health outcomes?

A. Answer *yes* to **"Before the illness or injury that brought you to the ED, did you need someone to help you on a regular basis?"**

B. Answer *no* to **"In general, do you see well?"**

C. Answer *yes* to **In general, do you have serious problems with your memory?**

D. Answer *yes* to **Do you take more than three medications every day?**

E. Answer *yes* to **Have you been hospitalized for one or more nights during the past 6 months?**

F. All of the above

#34

Answer: F

In addition, a 6th question asks about whether the patient has needed more help than usual to take care of themselves. The total score ranges from 0 to 6, and elderly patients are at high risk if they score 2 or greater on the questionnaire.

- *Samaras N, et al. Older patients in the emergency department: a review. Ann Emerg Med. 2010; 56:261-269. full text*

#35

You are seeing a violent, agitated, combative patient. It has become necessary to physically restrain the patient. TRUE statements about physical restraints include which of the following:

(Choose three answers.)

A. Initially, at least five staff members should restrain the patient.

B. Elevate the head of the bed.

C. The upper limb should be hyperabducted and extended.

D. The Joint Commission requires that a patient be assessed every 15 minutes after placement of restraints for signs of injury associated with the application of restraints.

#35

Answer: A, B, and D

Five staff members are necessary, one for each limb and a fifth to stand at the head of the bed to calm and explain the process to the patient. To avoid undermining the therapeutic relationship with the patient, the physician should not be part of this team. All patients are at risk for aspiration and the head of the bed should be slightly elevated. Restraint of an upper limb in the hyperabducted and extended position can cause peripheral nerve injury, so it should be repositioned at the patient's side as soon as adequate control of the patient is achieved.

- *Harwood-Nuss' Clinical Practice of Emergency Medicine 5th edition. 2010. Chapter 367: Legal Issues. 1684.*

#36

Which of the following patients is NOT at greater risk for sexual assault?

A. Age between 25-40 yo

B. Physically or mentally disabled

C. Homeless

D. Alcohol and drug users

E. College students

#36

Answer: A

The lifetime prevalence of sexual assault is 13 to 39% among women and 3% among men. Certain populations are at increased risk for sexual assault, including the physically or mentally disabled; homeless persons; persons who are gay, lesbian, bisexual, or transgendered; alcohol and drug users; college students; and persons under the age of 24 years.

- *Linden JA. Care of the adult patient after sexual assault. N Engl J Med. 2011 Sep 1; 365(9): 834-41. full text*

#37

Rape victims often present to the ED. If victims present within the time limit for evidence collection they should be referred to a local rape treatment center or offered the appropriate services if available via the ED. The time limit for evidence collection should not exceed:

A. 24-48 hours

B. 48-72 hours

C. 72-120 hours

D. One week

#37

Answer: C

Evaluation and treatment of sexual assault victims is time-intensive. In an ideal situation, a team should be available for consult through the ED. Teams generally include a medical provider, a trained sexual assault examiner, and a social worker or rape crisis counselor. Some regions have a sexual assault response team (SART) or a sexual assault nurse examiner (SANE). The members of the sexual assault teams are representatives from health care, forensics, the local rape crisis center, law enforcement and the prosecutor's office. The chain of evidence must be maintained during and after the examination. The sooner the examination occurs the better, with the upper time limit of 72-120 hrs varying by jurisdiction.

- *Linden JA. Care of the adult patient after sexual assault. N Engl J Med. 2011 Sep 1;365(9): 834-41. full text*

#38

Regarding sexual assault victims, which of the following statements is TRUE?

A. General body trauma is more frequent than genital trauma,

B. If an anogenital injury is not present, then it is unlikely for there to have been an assault.

C. Both of the above

D. Neither of the above

#38

Answer: A

It is not the responsibility of the medical providers to determine whether a sexual assault has occurred. The absence of anogenital injuries does not equate with absence of an assault. Although visual inspection only identifies anogenital injuries in less than half of victims, use of advance visualization techniques, such as colposcopy and toluidine blue staining increases identification rates to 53-84%. The rate of detection varies according to the age of the victim (more common if young or elderly), virginal status, degree of resistance, time from assault to examination, and the number of assailants.

- *Linden JA. Care of the adult patient after sexual assault. N Engl J Med. 2011 Sep 1; 365(9): 834-41. full text*

#39

All jurisdictions require mandatory reporting of which of the following:

(Choose three answers.)

A. Any rape

B. Weapons-related injuries in the competent adult

C. Assault of a child

D. Assault of an elderly person

E. Assault of a disabled person

#39

Answer: C, D, and E

Although some jurisdictions require mandatory reporting of rape or weapons-related injuries, this is not true for all jurisdictions. However, all jurisdictions require reporting the assault of a child or an elderly or disabled person.

- *Linden JA. Care of the adult patient after sexual assault. N Engl J Med. 2011 Sep 1; 365(9): 834-41. full text*

#40

Regarding the use of CT, which of the following is TRUE?

(Choose three answers.)

A. It is estimated that 1.5-2% of all cancers in the US are attributable to the radiation from CT.

B. Patient confidence in the accuracy of a medical evaluation that was limited to a physician-conducted history and physical evaluation was equal to an evaluation that included laboratory testing and CT.

C. Over 1/3 of patients think that CT delivers less radiation than 2-view chest X-rays.

D. Of patients who believed that they had never undergone a CT scan, over one-third had received a CT within the last 5 years.

#40

Answer: A, C, and D

Patient confidence was lowest for a medical evaluation that was limited to a physician conducted history and physical examination. The addition of lab testing and imaging resulted in a nearly 4-fold increase in confidence, with the highest confidence level in patients who were presented with the option of a CT. Patients are often not aware of the radiation exposure from a CT scan and may not even recall having advanced imaging.

- *Baumann BM, et al. Patient perceptions of computed tomographic imaging and their understanding of radiation risk and exposure. Ann Emerg Med. 2011 Jul; 58(1): 1-7.e2. full text*

#41

Regarding the use of CT, which of the following is TRUE?

A. Of patients who reported having had a CT scan documented in the electronic medical record, the mean number of scans in the previous 5 years was 5.4, with a range of 1 to 57 scans.

B. Patients accurately estimate the level of radiation received with CT imaging.

C. Both of the above

D. Neither of the above

#41

Answer: A

When participants were asked about their level of agreement with statements regarding radiation exposure and cancer risk statements, there was a low level of agreement with the statement “2 to 3 abdominal CTs give the same radiation exposure that survivors of Hiroshima received.” However, there was a modest level of agreement (45/100) with respect to the statement, “2 to 3 abdominal CTs over a person’s lifetime can increase the chances of cancer.” Patients also underestimate their previous imaging experiences, since 39% of patients who reported no previous CT 39% had one documented in the electronic medical record.

- *Baumann BM, et al. Patient perceptions of computed tomographic imaging and their understanding of radiation risk and exposure. Ann Emerg Med. 2011 Jul; 58(1): 1-7.e2. full text*

#42

Nontechnical skills are defined as the "cognitive, social and personal resource skills that complement technical skills, and contribute to safe and efficient task performance." Examples include communication and leadership. Which of the following nontechnical skills are linked to safety and error in the ED?

A. Supervising and providing feedback

B. Using assertiveness

C. Leadership

D. Closed loop communication

E. Situational awareness

F. All of the above

#42

Answer: F

All of the above nontechnical skills are associated with error and safety in the ED. Additional ones include anticipating and managing increasing workloads, maintaining high standards, and advanced decision making.

- *Flowerdew L, et al. Identifying nontechnical skills associated with safety in the ED: a scoping review of the literature. Ann Emerg Med. 2012 May; 59(5): 386-94. full text*

#43

Barriers to effective communication in the ED include which of the following?

A. Hierarchy – e.g., a resident is reluctant to question an attending

B. Noise in the department

C. Absence of somewhere to speak in private

D. All of the above

#43

Answer: D

All were barriers to communication. Additionally, closed-loop communication, in which the message is repeated to ensure correct transmission, may reduce errors.

- *Flowerdew L, et al. Identifying nontechnical skills associated with safety in the ED: a scoping review of the literature. Ann Emerg Med. 2012 May; 59(5): 386-94. full text*

#44

Workload management in the ED encompasses which of the following?

(Choose two answers.)

A. Lowering the noise level

B. Monitoring hand washing

C. Dealing with interruptions

D. Allocating tasks

#44

Answer: C and D

Workload management involves minimizing interruption, assigning tasks and roles for critical procedures, triaging and reassessing patient status, coordinating requests among teams and monitoring team activity.

- *Flowerdew L, et al. Identifying nontechnical skills associated with safety in the ED: a scoping review of the literature. Ann Emerg Med. 2012 May; 59(5): 386-94. full text*

www.ingramcontent.com/pod-product-compliance
Lightning Source LLC
Chambersburg PA
CBHW052306220526
45472CB00001B/4

* 9 7 8 1 9 8 0 4 9 2 1 0 8 *